INTERMITTENT FASTING

THE 21-DAY MEAL PLAN ON WHAT TO EAT AND THE THREE MOST COMMON MISTAKES WHICH PREVENT YOU FROM HAVING EXCELLENT HEALTH AND AN ENVIABLE PHYSIQUE. LOSE WEIGHT, SAVE MONEY, BE HAPPY

FABRICIUS MEAL

TABLE OF CONTENTS

INTRODUCTION 5

CHAPTER 1
BASICS OF INTERMITTENT FASTING 7

CHAPTER 2
THE TRUTH ABOUT INTERMITTENT FASTING 13

CHAPTER 3
INTERMITTENT FASTING AND AGING 21

CHAPTER 4
TYPES OF INTERMITTENT FASTING: 16/8 METHOD 25

CHAPTER 5
TYPES OF INTERMITTENT FASTING: 5:2 DIET 31

CHAPTER 6
TYPES OF INTERMITTENT FASTING: EAT STOP EAT 35

CHAPTER 7
BENEFITS OF INTERMITTENT FASTING 39

CHAPTER 8
21-DAY MEAL PLAN 45

CHAPTER 9
MOST COMMON MISTAKES 55

CHAPTER 10
BREAKFAST RECIPES 61

CHAPTER 11
LUNCH RECIPES 81

CHAPTER 12
DINNER RECIPES 101

CHAPTER 13
SNACK AND DESSERT RECIPES 121

CHAPTER 14
SMOOTHIE RECIPES 133

CHAPTER 15
MAINS RECIPES 153

CHAPTER 16
OTHER TYPES OF INTERMITTENT FASTING 173

CHAPTER 17
WHAT TO EAT WHILE INTERMITTENT FASTING 179

CHAPTER 18
INTERMITTENT FASTING AND WEIGHT LOSS 185

CHAPTER 19
INTERMITTENT FASTING TIPS FOR SUCCESS 191

CONCLUSION 195

INTRODUCTION

Intermittent Fasting is one of the in-demand health trends in the world. It has several positive effects on the body, such as enhanced health, weight loss, and a more simplified lifestyle. There have been countless studies to point out the benefits of Intermittent Fasting on the human body and mind.

It is an eating pattern where a person alternates between periods of eating and Fasting. Unlike other diet and meal plans, it doesn't specify what you should eat or avoid. Therefore, it isn't a diet in its strictest sense. It is more an eating pattern than a conventional diet. Though there are several intermittent methods, some of the most common are daily 16-hour fasts or 24-hour fasts twice a week.

Ancient food gathers and hunters didn't have the convenience of supermarkets and refrigerators. Food wasn't even available throughout the year. At times, they couldn't find anything to eat and went without food for days. The result: through evolution, the human body got accustomed to going without food for a long duration.

Fasting is what the body meant for. Eating more than 3-4 meals may not be as natural for the human body as Fasting because our bodies are inherently wired to go without food for longer periods. In addition to this, people also fasted for religious purposes. Many religions, such as Judaism, Buddhism, Hinduism, and Islam, practice going without food to clean the body and accomplish other spiritual/religious objectives.

Intermittent Fasting can be practiced in multiple ways, which involves splitting the week's 24-hour days into periods of eating and fasting. Different people pick different methods based on what is most convenient or suitable for them. During these fasting periods, you either eat little or nothing.

Intermittent Fasting is different from starvation in one important way. The one word for this difference is control. Starvation is the involuntary or forced absence from food. It is neither purposeful nor controlled. On the other hand, fasting is the voluntary withholding of meals for spiritual, religious, or health reasons. Food is available, but you deliberately choose not to consume it for the stipulated period.

It helps your body burn the excess stored fat. Contrary to what many people believe, Fasting, when done correctly, isn't unnatural or risky unless you suffer from specific medical conditions and have been advised to take caution. The problem is most people are not equipped with the knowledge to fast right. During Intermittent Fasting, our body exists in dual states, i.e., the feeding and fasting state. In the feeding state, our insulin levels soar, while in the fasting state, they plunge. The human body is forever, either storing or burning energy for meeting its energy needs. If the fasting duration is balanced by eating, the body's net weight doesn't increase.

Intermittent Fasting is not harmful. It is about maintaining body function cycles. Like a majority of people, if you are regularly involved in the process of eating, you will continue utilizing the newly incoming food energy without trying to burn what has already been accumulated.

Your body rarely goes into a fasting stage normally. It is one of the reasons people who practice Intermittent Fasting release their body fat without making any changes to how much and what they eat, or to their activities. While it is almost impossible to get your body into a fasting state within the standard fasting schedule, Intermittent Fasting can help fulfill your weight loss and other health goals.

CHAPTER 1

BASICS OF INTERMITTENT FASTING

Before trying out Intermittent Fasting, you have to find out whether it will work for you first. You have to determine if this eating pattern is appropriate for you first based on your present weight, lifestyle, body type, and health condition.

Note that even if it has plenty of benefits when done properly, like regulating your blood glucose, managing your body weight, gaining or maintaining lean muscle mass, and controlling blood lipids, it is not suitable for everyone. If you are still unsure, you may want to consult your doctor first.

Seek his advice and determine if your health will not get drastically affected by your decision to try Intermittent Fasting. In most cases, though, Intermittent Fasting seems to produce favorable and successful results for those who have the following or belong to any of the following:

- Have a history of monitoring food and calorie intake

- Has enough experience in terms of working out?

- Single or does not have children

- Have a supportive partner – someone who supports your decision to try IF

- Have a job that lets you have low-performance periods while adapting to a new eating pattern or plan

- Obtained a go-signal from their doctor to try IF

Intermittent Fasting can also greatly benefit those who intend to lose weight. Weight loss is one factor that encouraged most practitioners of this eating pattern to give it a try. Note that while some can significantly benefit from Intermittent Fasting, some should also avoid it as much as possible. It does not seem to work well for underweight or dealt with eating disorders in the past. You can still try it, though, but you have first to get the go-signal of a health professional.

It is not also highly recommended for those who are:

- Pregnant

- Suffering from chronic stress

- Have sleeping disorders

- Still new in terms of dieting and exercising

If you are still a beginner when it comes to dieting and working out, you may think that Intermittent Fasting is the best solution if your goal is to lose weight. However, you have to be wise enough to first address all possible nutritional deficiencies before experimenting with it fast. Start with a reliable nutritional platform if you are truly serious about doing Intermittent Fasting.

Also, remember that hunger is one of the major side effects of IF. It might even cause you to feel weak or lower the performance of your brain. Fortunately, these effects are usually only temporary. You will most likely experience them only while your body is still adapting to your new habits and eating patterns.

However, if you are suffering from a medical condition, seeking your doctor's advice is a must. Your doctor's opinion is even more important if you have diabetes, issues with regulating blood sugar, and low blood pressure.

One great thing about Intermittent Fasting is that it boasts of an outstanding safety profile. Fasting for a while will not cause you any harm, provided you are well-nourished and healthy overall. If you are still trying to figure out if you can significantly benefit from it, find out if you meet the following criteria:

- Your relationship with food is healthy.

- You can control your eating habits after breaking the fast.

- Your mental sharpness and productivity are not affected by fasting.

- You have good health overall.

- You have low or manageable stress levels.

The best way to determine if Intermittent Fasting is right for you is to try it for a while. If you still feel great even when you are fasting and discover that this approach is a more sustainable eating solution for you, you can view it as a truly powerful tool for your weight loss journey.

You can even use it to improve your health. Also, remember that there are certain factors that you have to focus on to maximize its benefits, including your workouts, sleeping patterns, and healthy eating habits.

What Body Type Can Benefit More From Intermittent Fasting?

As mentioned earlier, you can't expect Intermittent Fasting to work for everyone. The principles, patterns, and guidelines behind it do not suit all body types, too. There are three basic body types. There is the mesomorph, which is characterized by a solid and strong build.

Those who have this body type are usually neither underweight nor overweight. They seem to have rectangular body shapes and come with upright postures. Mesomorphs also have muscular legs and arms, muscular shoulders and chest, and even weight distribution.

Since mesomorphs do not often experience trouble eating whatever they want because they tend to lose weight easily, they may have an easier time crafting the perfect diet plan. However, they also tend to gain weight readily. In that case, Intermittent Fasting will surely work for them as this allows them to eat whatever they want during the eating window without worrying about their weight suddenly increasing.

Another body type that you have to be aware of is the endomorph. Fewer muscles and body fats often characterize the endomorph body type. This is the reason why those with this body type usually look soft and round. They also tend to put on pounds quickly and easily.

However, take note that being an endomorph does not necessarily mean you are already overweight. It is just that this body type tends to gain more weight quicker than the others. It is also quick and easy for endomorphs to increase their strength and build muscles.

If you have this body type, then a wise tip when it comes to dieting is to try reducing your carb intake. It is also advisable to increase your consumption of water and other healthy beverages for proper hydration. It is also important to note that endomorphs respond better to Intermittent Fasting than the other body types.

With that in mind, it is no longer surprising to see if IF is the go-to solution for endomorphs trying to lose weight or maintain a fit body. Intermittent Fasting also seems to work more effectively for endomorphs based on their metabolic rate.

The last body type is an ectomorph. You can see ectomorphs having a thinner body and lower weight and longer limbs. Compared to endomorphs, ectomorphs have a more accelerated metabolism. It is not easy for them to gain muscles, though they must perform specific exercises to improve their strength.

If you are an ectomorph, then know that your metabolism is different from endomorphs. In this case, Intermittent Fasting is not a good fit for your body type. It is the reason why it is not highly recommended for them. As far as body type is concerned, it seems to work more suitably for endomorphs.

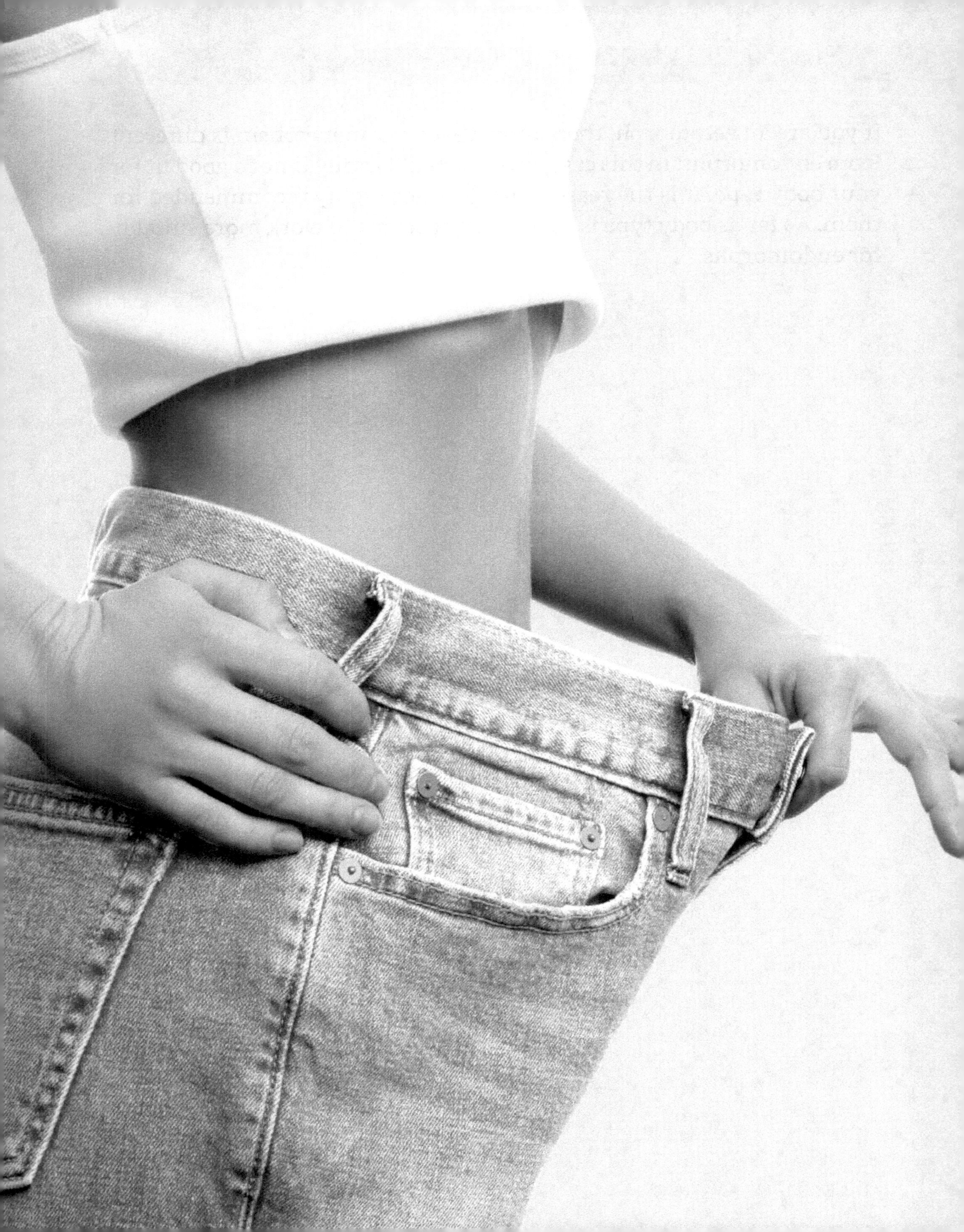

CHAPTER 2

THE TRUTH ABOUT INTERMITTENT FASTING

As vital as incorporating the fast into your lifestyle, you must care about what you want to get out of the fast as well. If you're unhappy with the results, it's doubtful you'll proceed with the lifestyle change you've initiated – all your energy will be wasted.

When looking at your goals, it's always advisable to use the SMART acronym:

- Specific

- Measurable

- Attainable

- Realistic

- Time-bound

An example of creating a SMART goal for your fast would work like this:

Specific – It needs to be made more specific. "I'm going to lose 10 pounds."

Measurable – How will you make sure you keep up with this? "I will quickly follow the 5 2 – pick Monday and Thursday as my fast days."

Attainable – Can this be done? Will it always be appropriate on Mondays and Thursdays? If you don't have a backup plan. "Wednesday is going to be my day of backup."

Realistic–Will you be able to stick to the calories of 500/600 on the 2 fast days? Would you eat healthily in the meantime?

Time-bound – You're going to want to keep an eye on your growth; you're heading to your target. "I'm going to weigh myself every week."

Making targets in this manner has been shown to have advantages and will help you achieve them. They are much more organized, they are possible, and they have nothing to hold you back. Print this knowledge and save it for you to use every day in a convenient location. Make yourself accountable.

Select The Best Time to Begin and the Most Effective Number of Meals to Suit This

Once you've figured out which program you want to follow, you'll need to figure out the most suitable hours to abstain from eating. You'll have to figure out the rest of it around your lifestyle and job.

Most fasts have a dictation about how many meals or treats you ought to eat every day. Others are more complex, leaving you with the alternative. Are you going to have one or two meals or five or six snacks? Due to the limited time and the way we usually work, most people choose to have up to 3 meals a day. Another approach is also more effective as it allows the body an ability to digest food more efficiently.

Decide on Foods to Include.

One of the most frequently asked fasting questions is, 'what can I eat?' Most diets don't say, but on the non-fasting days, it can be hard to know what 'eat as usual' entails. It is also a struggle on your fasting days to get the most out of your approved calories. You still want to get all you need to be able to work properly.

One of the most difficult things to train for a fast is getting past your food addiction. This may be something you don't even know you've got, but below is a list of signs to look for:

- Once you start eating certain foods, you end up eating more than expected.

- Although you're no longer hungry, you keep eating certain foods.

- You're eating to the point of feeling sick.

- You're concerned about not eating certain food types or about cutting down on certain food types.

- You go out of your way to get them when other things are not available.

- You eat particular foods so often or in such large quantities that you start eating food rather than studying, spending time with your family, or doing recreational activities.

- You avoid occupational or social environments in which certain foods are available due to fear of excessive consumption.

- Due to food and eating, you have problems working well at your job or college.

This condition can be troublesome and may compete with your dieting. It is usually associated with junk food, but can also be associated with carbohydrates, which will also cause problems with your speed. Below are some tips to help with this:

Eliminate processed foods–this kind of food is toxic and getting rid of it will only make you healthier.

Be careful–it will be challenging, of course, but you have to stick with it. The worst, but also the most rewarding, will be the first 48 hours.

Kill old habits–figure out when you eat badly and focus on that moment.

Increase the dosage slowly–don't do it too soon because you're going to have trouble.

Follow your nutritional needs–whatever you do, make sure you get all you need.

Have a cheat meal–don't starve yourself or find it more difficult to heal.

The diet will change depending on the days you don't eat and knowing that will benefit you in the long run. Exercising on an empty stomach has a lot of advantages. These include:

- A decrease in body fat

- Increased muscle tone

- Improved aerobic agility and consistency

- Potential to meet your fitness goals much faster

- Improvement in strength and sexual desire

- Stronger skin and decreased wrinkles

It is advised that you do interval training to get the most out of your exercise. You should have no trouble eating during the days you fast as long as you schedule your meals accordingly.

Remembering that fasting is not just about weight loss is very important. It can also help you build muscle mass–as the different diets included in this article have shown. Here are some tips on how to work out and build muscle as fast as you do:

- Late-night training sessions will help you manage your calories.

- During the recovery period, you will include protein and carbohydrates in your meal.

- Use the majority of your calories–approximately 60%–to help your body recover right after exercise.

- Eat about 20 percent of your daily calories before you work out to give you the strength you're going to need (while it's not essential as mentioned above, but should help build muscle mass).

- Do not exclude all fats–retain 'healthy' fats as a significant part of your diet.

- Try to eat by 5 am–it is recommended to eat early rather than later.

When building muscle isn't the ultimate goal, and fasting is more about burning fat, you might also try mixing aerobic workouts like biking, surfing, and athletics with one of the fasting diets. For the best results, it's advised to do at least some exercise alongside your fasting. Not only will you see your efforts perform even easier, but you will also begin to feel better and healthier earlier. You are free to choose a good exercise regime, as long as you do something.

The whole time you are fasting, there are things to keep in mind to keep you going. These include:

- One day at a time –don't worry about the future too much, just reflect on where you are.

- Goals–that is to say, always keep in mind your goals for inspiration.

- Rewards–reward yourself for achieving your goals. This will allow you to stay motivated. It need not be nutritional rewards; you should look for it outside the box.

- Nutrition –consider other nutrition-free remedies. You should retrain the brain just as much to enjoy healthy snacks. It only takes a little bit of time.

- Don't get caught up in the rules–it can be unhelpful to rely too much on the "do's and don'ts."

- Don't be too harsh on yourself–it's not the end of the world, even if you make mistakes, you will continue again at all times.

- Prepare–if you're committed to having something from all your food groups, your quick may be higher. You might just need to prepare your meals ahead of time.

- Get Started.

- Set your goal.

- Pick your target and keep it in mind. Choose a fasting plan based on your target and lifestyle.

- Make your promise.

- Make sure you stick to it once you set your mind to sporadic tempo. Do whatever it takes to make sure you're not going off track–even if that means telling someone and making sure they hold you accountable.

- Prepare and plan.

- Get it all in order. Make sure you're not holding anything back. Once the fasting is embedded in your daily routine, it will be smoother, but the first few days and weeks will be where the biggest challenge lies. Make sure you can relax as needed, but you have enough diversion to keep you going.

- Store.

- Make sure you have in your cupboards all the food you're going to need. You don't want to give up those excuses. This also refers to facilities for workouts.

Fluids to Take While Fasting

While fasting, only certain fluids can be consumed like; water, tea, and coffee (hot or iced) and homemade broth.

Water: The benefits of water cannot be overemphasized, so you must drink water frequently throughout the day when you fast. You can add:

- Slices of other fruits (never eat the fruit or consume fruit juice)

- Raw or unfiltered apple cider vinegar is better

- Lemon

- Himalayan salt

- Chia and ground flaxseed (mix one tablespoon in a cup of water)

- Sweetened powders or drops

Coffee: Consuming up to six cups of their caffeinated or decaffeinated coffee is allowed. Black coffee is preferable, but you are only allowed to add one tablespoon of certain fats to each cup of coffee taken. You can also have a change by taking unsweetened iced coffee. Brew your coffee and then refrigerate it or add ice cubes.

Herbal tea: There is no limit to the number of herbal teas you can consume during your fasting period. Some herbal teas can help suppress your appetite and lower your blood sugar levels.

Homemade Broth: It is normal if you experience some lightheadedness during the first few days of fasting. This is caused by dehydration and low electrolyte levels, and it can reduce by taking a good homemade broth. Both vegetable and broth made with meat, fish, or bones will work. Bone broth is very beneficial because it contains an essential ingredient called gelatin, which is very good for people with arthritis or other joint problems. There is no limitation of broth you can consume during the fasting day.

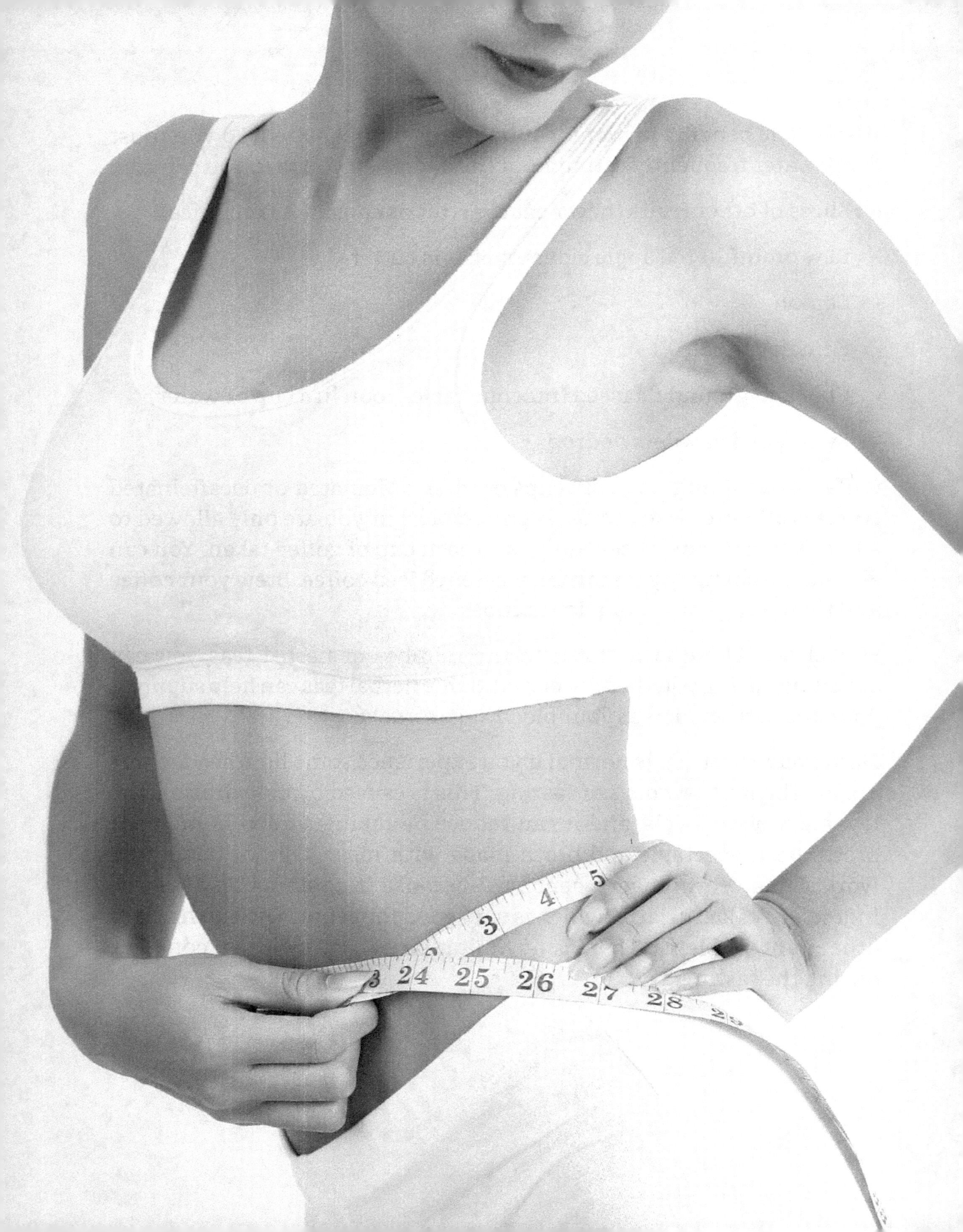

CHAPTER 3

INTERMITTENT FASTING AND AGING

Apart from weight and fat loss, Intermittent Fasting continues to gain traction because of its anti-aging benefits. Short term fasting protocols where calories are not consumed for at least 16 hours offer many independent benefits. These micro-fasts support metabolic health by lowering insulin levels, improving glycemic control, and controlling body weight.

Other fasting benefits include increased Brain Derived Neurotrophic Factor (BDNF) signaling in the brain, cardiovascular support, and lower risk of cancer recurrence. On the other hand, prolonged fasts of more than 48 hours stimulate different physiological changes that present unique fasting benefits to functional areas that include healthy aging, longevity, and immune strength.

Calorie restriction is one of the most efficient interventions for combating aging. Traditional calorie restriction usually reduces calories by between 20 and 40%. That is not recommended for performance and is not popular among biohackers because of the mental distraction that comes with it.

Fasting for Lifespan and Healthspan

Lifespan refers to the duration of time we live. On the other hand, the healthspan is the length of time you're functional and healthy and not just alive. Calorie restriction influences and is valuable for both healthspan and lifespan. Unfortunately, it's common to focus on the life span's detriment to the quality of your life within longevity and aging space. On the contrary, the length of time you're functional and healthy is linked to a higher quality of life. Healthspan can be mediated by various factors that include dietary interventions and social interactions. It's more valuable to emphasize healthspan than lifespan.

Damage Accumulation vs. Programmed Aging

There's a debate between the importance of damage accumulations and programmed aging. Even then, it's essential to recognize the complexity of the human system in understanding physiological debates. Programmed aging is all about the changes in the manner in which genes are expressed in aging. Some of these changes are over expressed, while others are under-expressed. Damage accumulation is characterized by mitochondrial and cellular damage over time. Both damage accumulation and programmed aging occur at the cellular level, each amplifying the other's effects. Here are three ways Intermittent Fasting helps you to live longer:

Hormesis

Evidence has proven that regular Intermittent Fasting will help cells become more resilient to any form of cellular stress. Cellular resilience is caused by the hormesis process, which simply describes the biological responses to stress. A little stress from daily fasting can help avoid negative effects and instead produce positive biological responses that increase resilience to oxidative stress.

Intermittent Fasting increases ketones

Your body is deprived of glucose from the consumption of protein and carbohydrates when in the fasted state. The body prefers to draw energy from glucose, but it changes when you fast. It breaks down fat stored in the liver that turns into ketones, an available source of energy in the absence of glucose. Ketones are shuttled to the mitochondria, where they're used as fuel for muscles, hearts, and brains. Even then, certain parts of your body cannot utilize ketones and only require glucose. This glucose is supplied by breaking down protein and fat glycerol through gluconeogenesis. Ketones have some anti-aging benefits. Take the example of Alzheimer's disease.

Fasting triggers autophagy

The process of autophagy will slow down the ability to recycle cells that are under stress. Fasting activates and increases autophagy, which slows down the rate of aging as the body is primed to combat stress. When you're fasting and your insulin levels drop effectively, increasing autophagy.

Overall, Intermittent Fasting is a simple intervention that has profound benefits that go beyond weight loss. When you eat within a defined window every day, you activate several anti-aging pathways. Ultimately, you also must take into account other factors like healthy eating and proper hydration.

CHAPTER 4

TYPES OF INTERMITTENT FASTING: 16/8 METHOD

One of the reasons many people worldwide are seeing success with Intermittent Fasting is that there are a variety of methods that have been developed through study and experience to meet a range of health desires and achieve any number of personal wellness goals. This will give a closer look at the most popular, studied, and proven-to-be-effective method of Intermittent Fasting, how they work, and who they work best for.

16/8 Method

The 16/8 method of fasting is, without a doubt, one of the most popular methods of Intermittent Fasting around. This is the easiest way to achieve your weight loss goals that you have been pondering for months.

This method doesn't require a lot of planning. It is super easy to follow, and the results visible from an early stage. Whether you have been struggling with a few extra kilograms or looking for a complete transformation, this method is for you.

This method entails a fasting period of 16 hours, during which no calories are consumed in any way. No solid or fluids containing calories are allowed. During the sixteen hours, you may, however, drink much water as you need. This is followed by eight hours of calorie consumption. Once this cycle is complete, you may repeat this as often and as you wish. Remember, hydrate, and eat nutrient-rich foods to sustain your daily activity levels.

Intermittent Fasting aids in weight loss by creating an opportunity for calorie restriction. You will lose weight when you expend more energy than you consume daily.

The beauty of the 16/8 method lies in the fact that you spend a great deal of your fasting period sleeping. This prevents you from indulging and distracts you from the fact that you may feel a little hungry. When there is no fresh and consumed nutrient available, the body has to mobilize energy sources stored in the body. For the body to be able to do this, it needs active energy. Therefore, it uses some energy to reach the stored glucose and fat in your cells.

This has two significant effects. Firstly, it utilizes all of the carbohydrates available and prevents these carbohydrates from being stored as fat. Secondly, it mobilizes fat stored in your cells, which in essence leads to the process of fat burning. The combination of decreased fat storage and increased fat burning leads to the desired fat loss effect.

Intermittent Fasting, in addition to the above mentioned, has a boosting effect on the metabolism. Studies have shown that Intermittent Fasting affects your appetite and has a stabilizing impact on hormones that control your fat-burning rate.

Why the 16/8 method is so effective

The 16/8 method is one of the most effective ways of Intermittent Fasting. The main reason for this is that it is one of the easiest methods to get into. It is simple and doesn't require a lot of preparation.

Combine fasting with comfort and the words "eat whatever you like for eight hours," and you have a winning method. The greatest part of fasting usually takes place while you are sleeping. This acts as a distraction for the hunger pain that you might be feeling. Create a busy schedule for yourself, sleep a little, and skip breakfast. It is lunchtime, and your sixteen hours fast has ended.

This way of fasting is one of the least restrictive types. It doesn't have many rules, and it still creates great results. This method can be adjusted to fit your lifestyle and activity level. This method is for everyone.

How to prepare it

The most important part of your fast is not necessarily the eating plan or the time frame, but rather the preparation for the process. Make sure to prepare yourself for the process ahead. Understand what is expected of you and how it works.

Plan out your days. This process may be physically and mentally challenging. If you step into this process with an open mind and a proper plan, you will succeed.

The important thing to consider is that fasting is not a diet. Fasting can and should become part of your life. Use this as a test run to learn new habits and change your lifestyle for the better.

Another key point to consider is that good things take time. Give yourself a few weeks to adapt. Don't give up too soon, it will become easier, and you will see results.

Physical preparation

During your physical preparation, you first need to decide within which times you will consume your calories. Here you need to consider your schedule; what time you wake up, when you usually have lunch and, what time you go to bed. You need an eight-hour slot in which you can comfortably consume food.

Most commonly, people choose to skip the first meal of the day. For example, you consume your last meal at 7 pm on Thursday, and this means that your following meal and first meal of Friday will take place at 11 am. If you choose to do this for a prolonged period, this will be your window of eating. You will be able to consume food between 11 am and 7 pm daily.

You may choose for your last meal at 8 pm, which would mean your first meal would take place at 12 pm. Your daily eating window, therefore, is 12 pm - 8 pm daily. Consider your schedule and choose a convenient time.

If you prefer to have breakfast, you can consume your breakfast meal at any time as long as you stick to an eight-hour window. If you choose to have breakfast at 8 am, your last meal will take place at 4 pm on the same day. This will then serve as your daily window for the time that you choose to follow this process.

After deciding on your eating menu, you need to stock up on a few healthy and nutritional foods. Ensure that you have food around to keep yourself from reaching for unhealthy options when you feel starving after your fast. Plan what you would like your first meal to be.

If you have the time and don't mind eating leftovers, prepare a few meals in advance. Make sure they are nutritious and available when you feel hungry. This will keep you from overeating and curb the cravings.

Mental preparation

Fasting can take a mental toll on you, especially if this is your first time trying something like this. Mental preparation will help you get through this with ease.

The most important thing is to have a goal in mind. Write it down and check yourself. Visualizing your progress will help you stay positive on tough days.

Know what you are getting yourself into. Understand before embarking on this journey that it may be challenging, and you may fail a few times.

Brush it off and try again. One small setback doesn't mean that you can't reach your goal. Keep moving forward.

Find something or someone that motivates you and tell them about your journey. Get a friend to join you. You can keep each other accountable, struggle together, and be each other's motivation. All the good things in life take time. Be patient.

CHAPTER 5

TYPES OF INTERMITTENT FASTING: 5:2 DIET

The 5:2 diet is a calorie-restrictive diet that includes intermittent and modified fasting. Five days on a diet, you eat what you want (the feed days), and for two days, you do a modified fast (the fast days). The two days of modified fasting should not be done consecutively.

If you want to commit to the 5:2 diet, make sure to see your doctor first. There are some people that fasting can harm like pregnant women, people who have compromised immunity, those that are already underweight, children, teenagers, and people with a history of eating disorders.

The Fasting Days

Before you start the 5:2 diet, you need to decide which two non-consecutive days of the week you want to designate as fast days. These days will include modified fasting, where you will cut your calorie intake to about one-quarter of the calories you would typically consume in a day.

Women are allowed to consume 500 calories on fast days

Men are allowed to consume 600 calories on fast days

Dr. Michael Mosley chose to fast on Mondays and Thursdays. He strategically wanted workdays in which he was less likely to think about food.

On the last days, he would typically split his allowable 600 calories between breakfast and dinner. He would typically have breakfast at about 7:30 am, which would consist of a couple of scrambled eggs and ham, about 300 calories.

Throughout the day, he would drink lots of water, black tea, and black coffee until evening.

At 7:30 pm he would eat a 300-calorie dinner that consisted of lots of fresh vegetables and a slice of salmon. By modifying fast, he allowed his body to have approximately two 12-hour periods of fasting in a 24-hour day. Mosley believes this is the most manageable and straightforward way of modified fasting on fast days.

You can adjust your eating on fast days to whatever works best with your schedule, but studies have shown that a long stretch of fasting can be more effective than breaking your 500 or 600 calories down into a couple of meals and a small snack in between.

Fasting for prolonged periods (more than 12-14 hours) can be harmful to your health and should only be done under medical supervision. Short bursts of Intermittent Fasting, as suggested on the 5:2 diet is ideal and compliment your health. Be careful not to overdo fasting. Only do what is recommended by the 5:2 food.

For five days on a diet, you are allowed to eat whatever you want. This is where most people begin to question the effectiveness of the 5:2 diet. Why? Because it doesn't seem reasonable to be able to eat what you want and still lose weight.

Who Can Do the 5:2 Intermittent Fasting Diet Plan?

Similar to all other diet techniques out there, this one should also be carefully undertaken. It is a simple control over one's food intake, but it still holds risks if you are unhealthy or suffering from a condition. Pregnant women and nursing mothers are one of the risk groups who should avoid the 5:2 diet plan. It is because an expectant mother has to provide nutrients for herself and the unborn baby she is carrying. The fetus faces malnutrition during this stage and can cause complications in the pregnancy. It also results in dizziness, which could lead to a physical injury that could also cause pregnancy problems.

People who have type-1 diabetes should also avoid this diet because it brings about profound changes across the blood glucose levels during the fasting day. Diabetics already have a low insulin level within their bodies to regulate sudden shifts in glucose concentrations. So, it is highly advised against for them to use the 5:2 diet plan.

Another populous that should stay clear of the 5:2 diet plan are people who have a chronic or acute medical condition. In this case, it is easier for a medical specialist to identify whether you can or cannot follow this diet plan. They might help you plan out the perfect diet plan or modify the 5:2 policy to better suit your needs without risking your life.

Some people argue that cutting calories so drastically can be harmful to the body. However, that is not the case, and unless you are part of the small risk group stated above, you can follow this diet plan. In reality, fasting has proven to aid the body. It helps the body repair itself and cleans out all of its circulatory systems. The health benefits show how effective the 5:2 diet can be for improving your body's overall condition. You should not be worried about the drastic reduction in calories during the fast day because our bodies are designed to deal with this situation. 5:2 dieting has already proven to be as effective as regular dieting techniques and a higher success rate.

Risks and other precautions

The diet plan is simple and relatively strong, but it is still wise for you to be careful, especially during the first few fasting days. Most people find that hunger pangs are the only problem that they face during the fast day. Most of them confirm that they do not feel dizzy or lethargic during the day and that after some time, the hunger pangs also subside. Be careful about what you do during the initial weeks and monitor how your body reacts to the diet plan.

You can and should do some mild exercise during the fast days as it helps the body burn the stored fat. This brings more energy to your muscles and makes you feel more active. However, extremely strenuous exercise must be avoided during fast days. You should always listen to your body and stop when you start to feel pain or get too tired to continue. You should not try to push your body beyond its limits while you are fasting. And even though you exercise during the fast day, you cannot add calories to your 500 or 600 Kcal limit as a trade-in for your workout.

Another risk associated with diet plans is the possibility of developing eating disorders. Be mindful of your eating habits to stop at once if you feel you are losing control. Eating disorders can range from not eating enough to overeating. Eating all 2000 calories in one sitting is also considered an eating disorder and should be a sign for you to stop your diet and seek professional assistance.

This 5:2 diet plan is so simple and easy to follow that they find it pointless to keep their bodies healthy only because they have achieved the desired weight loss.

CHAPTER 6

TYPES OF INTERMITTENT FASTING: EAT, STOP, EAT

The Eat Stop Eat is not a daily fasting program, and it mostly encourages you to fast just once per week. The fasting period, in this case, would be only 24 hours, which might sound a bit scary for some of you out there

The 24-hour fast is one of the most popular programs practiced by different people worldwide. It was developed by Brad Pilon, who had the bright idea to name this program very simple: Eat Stop Eat.

There are plenty of specialists and people who can agree that this program is the easiest one, and perhaps it should be the first Intermittent Fasting program to be tried by beginners. Some people might be thinking of trying more IF programs, but you need to ease into Intermittent Fasting; to take it slow because you will be able to deal a lot easier with possible symptoms like hunger, headaches, and dizziness.

The Eat Stop Eat program is perhaps the most accessible and popular method for most Intermittent Fasting enthusiasts. Some people like to fast entirely for one day per week, every once in a while. Others are more ambitious and might want to try the 24 hours fast twice or three times a week. This program doesn't require any scheduling or special rules. You only have one control: choose the day you want to fast.

Just like any other Intermittent Fasting program, this one doesn't mention anything about a particular meal plan, and you can eat whatever you want, as long as you respect the only rule that you have. Suppose you plan to try this program (or any Intermittent Fasting). In that case, you might need to take it easy with the calorie intake, as you probably want to lose some weight, or even experience some other health benefits of Intermittent Fasting.

One of the best advantages of the 24 hours fast is that you have plenty of feeding days, so, in other words, your body will not lack any macronutrients to function properly and to be energized. Like all the other Intermittent Fasting programs, the best way is to work out on an empty stomach. Some people would prefer just a few exercises to be in shape (like ab crunches or push-ups), while others prefer to jog, swim, or work out at the gym early in the morning.

You still need to enter the fasted state (daily) to find the best time for working out. So why not have a ten-hour eating period? Let's say from 9 am to 7 pm. This doesn't sound too harsh. You can still have three main meals per day, and you can also enter the fasted state to work out daily, immediately after 7 am. You can head over to the gym early in the morning if you have the last meal at 7 pm, and start training after 7 am. Usually, a typical training session should not last longer than 75 minutes, so this can give you plenty of time to shower, have a consistent breakfast (after 9 am), and get to work.

But what about the fast day? Can you work out during that day? It's highly recommendable to work out during that day. Training can give you the energy boost you need for the day, plus you will feel a lot better and more agile, as you will not feel the fat tissue slowing you down.

When you are on this program, it's better to find a way to work all of your muscle groups. You can jog to burn calories, but it will not train all your muscles. However, swimming does, and you have plenty of equipment at your local gym to work out all the muscles of your body. Swimming can be an enjoyable way to get a lean mass that you've always wanted, but if you're going to increase in size and build muscles, you will need to work out at the gym.

CHAPTER 7

BENEFITS OF INTERMITTENT FASTING

There are many benefits you can gain once you choose to eat the Intermittent Fasting way. When you embrace the irregular fasting lifestyle, regardless of what style of this diet, you decide to eat, you will gain many incredible benefits. While some of these benefits are true to other diets, they are not nearly as convenient or healthy to achieve. Many diets require specific calorie counting, meal plans, or food choices to be considered valid. With the Intermittent Fasting diet, you do not have to worry so much about any of that. As a result, it is a much more flexible and enjoyable diet that allows you to continue eating.

In addition to convenience and flexibility, there several other benefits that you stand to gain. From a reduced likelihood of contracting diseases and illnesses to supporting you in healing from injuries at a higher speed, there is plenty to look forward to from the Intermittent Fasting diet.

Healthier Way to Lose Weight

Intermittent Fasting is a healthier way for people to lose weight. As a result of this diet's flexibility, you are still able to continue consuming everything healthy for you. Any dietary considerations you may need to accommodate can quickly be taken into consideration and accounted for with Intermittent Fasting. This makes it easy and effortless when it comes to losing weight.

Unlike other diets, there are no restricting calories or starving yourself with the Intermittent Fasting diet. You will not experience any sensations of hunger or feeling as though you are not getting enough. Whereas other foods are often not maintained for long, resulting in unhealthy practices of "yo-yo" dieting, Intermittent Fasting can be. This means that the food is not only healthier but also more sustainable.

When you are eating the Intermittent Fasting diet, you can look forward to losing fat specifically. This diet supports you in letting go of unwanted fats in your body that may be stubborn and resistant to other foods. Intermittent Fasting is both healthier and more effective in supporting you with reaching your weight loss goals.

When your cells have an easier time restoring themselves, and your body is exposed to less stress, you have an easier time healing faster. This means that any time you place a physical strain on your body, you can look forward to treating less from that experience.

This is beneficial for many reasons. You can increase your health faster when you heal more quickly. Activities such as working out and lifting weights require your body to take some downtime to heal in between. Any time you are seeking to increase your muscular strength, you will experience ripping in your muscles. Then, the muscle tissue heals and grows back in a higher quantity. This is what leads to muscle growth. It is also what leads to pain after working out.

When you eat according to the Intermittent Fasting diet, your ability to heal from this type of damage is improved. This means that you can gain muscle faster and without harming your overall health.

In addition to intentional healing required after activities such as working out, you will also have an easier time healing from other physical ailments. For example, if you endure an accidental injury, your body will have an easier time healing it than if you were in ill health.

Because your body has an improved ability to repair cells, you can look forward to healing much quicker from any injury that you might experience.

You Can Maintain a More Youthful Appearance

Improved cellular repairs and gene expression are great for healing, but it is also great for maintaining a youthful vitality. When these functions improve for you, your body's ability to maintain a healthier skin, hair, nails, and other bodily features is also improved. This means that you can maintain a more youthful appearance by adjusting your diet and eating the Intermittent Fasting way.

In addition to actually looking more youthful, you can enjoy the experience of feeling younger, too. People who eat the Intermittent Fasting diet report feeling greater levels of energy. As a result, they can start enjoying life with a greater vitality about them. This means that you can enjoy all of the activities that you have been missing as a result of low energy and ill health, like dancing and spending time enjoying life with your loved ones.

Lowers Your Risk of Contracting Diseases

When your immune system is operating optimally, and your entire bodily functions are improved, you can enjoy the lowered risk of contracting diseases. As you already know, diseases like type 2 diabetes, Alzheimer's, and cancer have been prevented by the Intermittent Fasting diet. However, this diet can also support you in preventing other potential diseases.

Eating the Intermittent Fasting diet has proven to level out blood pressure, reduce bad cholesterol, lower inflammatory markers, and lower blood sugar levels that you can look forward to having better heart health. You also work toward preventing heart disease by eating this way.

Reduced instances of inflammation markers also mean that the Intermittent Fasting diet can also support you in preventing or curing symptoms of diseases like fibromyalgia. They can also help you heal from chronic fatigue syndrome and other conditions that are typically related to poor inner health.

Reduces Inflammation and Physical Stress

The Intermittent Fasting diet is known to eliminate free radicals from your body. This means that you are less likely to experience chronic inflammation and physical stress based on nutrition and nourishment.

For many people, chronic inflammation and physical stress derived from nourishment can be the root cause of many physical symptoms. Often, people go undiagnosed yet continue to experience frustrating symptoms like pain, swelling, headaches, and metabolic issues when they experience chronic inflammation. It can lead to frustration, hopelessness, and anger when it comes to trying to resume a healthy and active lifestyle. Intermittent Fasting may help you overcome these symptoms if they are being caused by chronic inflammation or physical stress.

May Extend Your Lifespan

Intermittent Fasting has shown in some studies that it may be able to extend your lifespan. Many people find themselves living shorter lives with poorer quality of life as a result of poor health. Disease and illness kill far more people each year than actual old age or natural causes do. Using the Intermittent Fasting diet may help you prevent these illnesses and diseases so that you can live a longer, healthier, natural life.

The Intermittent Fasting diet was tested in lab rats but not yet tested in humans. Some studies showed that the rats lived as much as 83% longer than those who did not fast. Despite this specific evidence not yet been tested on humans, there is plenty of evidence suggesting that the factors that prevent longer and healthier lives can be avoided with

Intermittent Fasting. Thus, we can assume that Intermittent Fasting may indeed support humans in living longer and healthier lives, too.

Boosts Your Immune System

Intermittent Fasting can also get you to look forward to having an improved immune system. This is due to reduced physical stress, increased cellular reparation abilities, weight loss, and other benefits that you gain from Intermittent Fasting.

Your boosted immune system will be supportive in preventing you from experiencing long-term health conditions such as various illnesses and diseases. It will also help you prevent the contraction of less dangerous diseases such as the common cold and influenza. You can enjoy life and spend less time being sick.

CHAPTER 8

21-DAY MEAL PLAN

Fasting is meant to be modified to fit your life. You should not have to turn your personal and social life upside down to fit a specific style of Intermittent Fasting. Short-term progress is relevant, real success always comes in the medium to long term and keep that in mind as you venture forward on this fasting journey.

To cover meals plans for the different types of fasts, start asking yourself these essential questions:

What time of the day do you choose most of your eating?

Do you prefer frequent, more modest fasts or infrequent, longer ones?

There are many alternative strategies to ensure that you arrive at a style of fasting or possibly a combination of methods that works best for you.

FASTING TIME	16 HOURS
EATING TIME	8 HOURS
CALORIES ALLOWED DURING FAST	NONE
MEALS PER DAY	2 MEALS PER DAY, SNACK OPTIONAL NOTE: BEGINNERS MAY CHOOSE TO FAST ONLY ON ALTERNATING DAYS

The meal plans provided for 16:8 fasters will only include lunch and dinner to facilitate the 16-hour fasting period.

Depending on your usual routine, you may choose to incorporate a snack either in between or after these meals. You can increase the serving size of the meal, especially during the first week or two. Feel free to replace any lunch recommendations with leftovers from dinner.

Remember, the key component here is the 16-hour period from your last bite one day to your first bite the next.

DAYS	BREAKFAST	LUNCH	DINNER
1	FAST	COLLARD GREENS AND BACON	AROMATIC ZUCCHINI NOODLES SOUP
2	FAST	AROMATIC ZUCCHINI NOODLES SOUP	PIZZA
3	FAST	ASPARAGUS AND SRIMP MIX	PUMPKIN SOUP

DAYS	BREAKFAST	LUNCH	DINNER
4	Fast	Pumpkin Soup	Tofu Pesto Peppers
5	Fast	Chicken and Broccoli Casserole	Garlic Broccoli
6	Fast	Garlic Broccoli	Lobster Bisque
7	Fast	Lemon Chicken	Parmesan Tomatoes
8	Fast	Parmesan Tomatoes	Halloumi Salad
9	Fast	Tasty Thai Beef	Tomato Soup
10	Fast	Spaghetti Squash	Herbed Salmon Fillets
11	Fast	Herbed Salmon Fillets	Tangy Fennel Salad
12	Fast	Collard Greens and Bacon	Spinach Cheese Pie
13	Fast	Spinach Cheese Pie	Baked Cheese Asparagus
14	Fast	Baked Cheese Asparagus	Tomato Kebabs
15	Fast	Italian-Inspired Chicken Breast	Butter Glazed Carrots
16	Fast	Ultimate Corn on the Cob	Gratifying Meatloaf
17	Fast	Gratifying Meatloaf	Aromatic Zucchini Noodles Soup
18	Fast	Aromatic Zucchini Noodles Soup	Baked Cheese Asparagus

DAYS	BREAKFAST	LUNCH	DINNER
19	Fast	Hearty Lemon & Garlic Pork	Tofu Pesto Peppers
20	Fast	Tofu Pesto Peppers	Juicy Brussels Sprouts
21	Fast	Butter Glazed Carrots	Pizza

5:2

FASTING DAYS PER WEEK	2
NORMAL EATING DAYS PER WEEK	5
CALORIES ALLOWED DURING FASTING DAYS	<800
MEALS PER DAY	ALL CALORIES ARE EATEN WITHIN 1 TO 8 HOURS ON FASTING DAYS, EITHER IN ONE SITTING ON FASTING DAYS OR IN TWO SMALLER MEALS

On regular days, 5:2 fast will follow the standard plans of three meals per day for a given week.

You may choose to eat differently and focus on snacks or smaller meals on fasting days, in which case some additional effort is required to ensure you stay within the 500- to 800-calorie range. You might, for example, choose to eat one large meal in the 500- to 800-calorie range, or you might have one moderately sized meal and one snack of about 300 calories to land you in that range.

For days you are not fasting, feel free to replace any lunch recommendation with leftovers from dinner.

DAYS	BREAKFAST	LUNCH	DINNER
1	Breakfast Quesadillas	Butter Glazed Carrots	Pizza
2	Fast	Pizza	Juicy Brussels Sprouts
3	Swiss and Pear Omelet	Spaghetti Squash	Herbed Salmon Fillets
4	Ham and Asparagus Casserole	Herbed Salmon Fillets	Tangy Fennel Salad
5	Fast	Tasty Thai Beef	Tomato Soup
6	Blueberry Compote and Yogurt	Tomato Soup	Aromatic Zucchini Noodles Soup
7	Pineapple Coconut Deluxe Smoothie	Aromatic Zucchini Noodles Soup	Tomato Kebabs
8	Blueberry Scones	Tomato Kebabs	Lobster Bisque
9	Fast	Ultimate Corn on the Cob	Gratifying Meatloaf
10	Mini Quiche	Hearty Lemon & Garlic Pork	Tofu Pesto Peppers
11	Banana Pudding	Tofu Pesto Peppers	Juicy Brussels Sprouts
12	Fast	Lemon Chicken	Parmesan Tomatoes
13	Cherry and Almond Breakfast Cookies	Parmesan Tomatoes	Halloumi Salad

DAYS	BREAKFAST	LUNCH	DINNER
14	Sweet Potato Pancakes	Collard Greens and Bacon	Tomato Soup
15	Raspberry Coconut Smoothie	Chicken and Broccoli Casserole	Garlic Broccoli
16	Fast	Italian-Inspired Chicken Breast	Tangy Fennel Salad
17	Peanut Butter Energy Cookies	Tangy Fennel Salad	Aromatic Zucchini Noodles Soup
18	Sunflower Cookies	Spinach Cheese Pie	Baked Cheese Asparagus
19	Fast	Baked Cheese Asparagus	Ultimate Corn on the Cob
20	Blueberry Compote and Yogurt	Ultimate Corn on the Cob	Tofu Pesto Peppers
21	Apple Walnut Loaf	Tofu Pesto Peppers	Herbed Salmon Fillets

FASTING DAYS PER WEEK	3 TO 4 NOTE: FULL DAY OF FASTING ON ALTERNATING DAYS
NORMAL EATING DAYS PER WEEK	3 TO 4 NOTE: FULL DAY OF FASTING ON ALTERNATING DAYS
CALORIES ALLOWED DURING FAST	NONE
MEALS PER DAY	3 MEALS PER DAY ON EATING DAYS, SNACK OPTIONAL, NONE ON FASTING DAYS NOTE: BECAUSE ALTERNATING DAYS CAN MEAN YOU FAST EITHER 3 OR 4 DAYS IN A WEEK, YOU CAN ALTER THE DIFFICULTY OF THE FAST BY CHOOSING WHETHER THE FIRST DAY OF THE WEEK IS A FASTING OR EATING DAY

Alternate-day fasters will eat freely one day and fast the next. On free-eating days, you can use the following meal plan provided. You may choose to incorporate additional snacks or double the serving size of specific recipes as your hunger dictates.

For days you are not fasting, feel free to replace any lunch recommendation with leftovers from dinner.

DAYS	BREAKFAST	LUNCH	DINNER
1	Apple Walnut Loaf	Ultimate Corn on the Cob	Tofu Pesto Peppers
2	Fast	Fast	Fast
3	Sunflower Cookies	Spinach Cheese Pie	Baked Cheese Asparagus
4	Fast	Fast	Fast
5	Cherry and Almond Breakfast Cookies	Lemon Chicken	Parmesan Tomatoes
6	Fast	Fast	Fast
7	Mini Quiche	Hearty Lemon & Garlic Pork	Tangy Fennel Salad
8	Pineapple Coconut Deluxe Smoothie	Tasty Thai Beef	Tomato Soup
9	Fast	Fast	Fast
10	Blueberry Scones	Hearty Lemon & Garlic Pork	Juicy Brussels Sprouts
11	Fast	Fast	Fast
12	Breakfast Quesadillas	Chicken and Broccoli Casserole	Halloumi Salad
13	Fast	Fast	Fast
14	Ham and Asparagus Casserole	Collard Greens and Bacon	Aromatic Zucchini Noodles Soup

DAYS	BREAKFAST	LUNCH	DINNER
15	Banana Pudding	Tasty Thai Beef	Garlic Broccoli
16	Fast	Fast	Fast
17	Swiss and Pear Omelet	Lemon Chicken	Baked Cheese Asparagus
18	Fast	Fast	Fast
19	Sweet Potato Pancakes	Hearty Lemon & Garlic Pork	Gratifying Meatloaf
20	Fast	Fast	Fast
21	Raspberry Coconut Smoothie	Italian-Inspired Chicken Breast	Tangy Fennel Salad

CHAPTER 9

Intermittent Fasting might sound like a simple concept, but with only one simple mistake, all your weight loss efforts can go down the drain. One reason why most women fail to attain their desired results is that they have trouble adjusting to the plan. For many women, Intermittent Fasting is vastly different from the diet that they have followed in the past. Look at some mistakes which must be avoided at all costs:

Consuming a High Amount of Carbohydrates Daily

Carbohydrates are one of the major sources of energy for your body, and the amount and type of carbohydrates you consume determines your body's glucose level. When you eat lots of carbs, mainly processed ones, your blood glucose level tends to reach a higher level on a regular or daily basis.

But when you fast the other day for 10-12 hours straight, then there's a significant drop in your glucose level, which can put major strains on your brain and nervous system. This can also make you feel grouchy, irritable, or moody. It is thus advised to eat less carb-based food and consume more vegetables and fats instead.

Not Caring About the Eating Window

If you're fasting for long hours like 16, 20, or more hours, you should include an eating window where you could gobble up some snacks or drinks. Fasting for such long hours could leave you too weak.

But having an eating window is not enough. Keep the window short and be careful about what you eat during this time, for example, five minutes. Have some crackers, fruits, sandwiches, or a cup of coffee.

Eating Without Realizing It

When you're on IF, to get the best results out of it, you should strictly restrict yourself from consuming anything, water being an exception. Beverages like coffee and diet soda can increase appetite, making it difficult for you to continue with your fasting.

Binge eating

When you fast for 16 hours straight, it's human nature to devour on whatever your eyes see first. But if you're practicing Intermittent Fasting for the sole purpose of losing weight, you should closely monitor your food consumption after fasting.

IF works by using up the extra fat stored in your body as energy. If you replenish that by consuming more calories than you lost, then your entire IF will be considered a failure. As a rule of thumb, don't rush to KFC or McDonald's to break your fasting. But you can have lots of fruits, vegetables, complex carbs, and mildly processed food.

Not Drinking Enough Water

While consuming calories or drinking any form of beverages is prohibited, drinking water is encouraged since it has no calories. As you're aware, the stomach releases an acid that aids in the digestion of our food.

When you're fasting, your stomach remains empty for a long time, causing acid to develop and accumulate. Accumulation of large amounts of these acids can cause stomach complications and irritations. Water prevents this situation by diluting the acid, thus keeping you focused on your Intermittent Fasting.

Not Eating Enough

One of the mistakes women make is they don't eat enough after their fasting hours. The main job of Intermittent Fasting is to use up the excess energy stored in the fat cells, not to deprive you of essential nutrients.

Additionally, when you don't eat for an extended time, you lose hunger and become less hungry (this is your body's way of fighting back). This is why some people tend to under-eat while some overeat. Thus, after your IF routine, make sure to refuel yourself with nutritious food like fruits, nuts, and vegetables - not with junk food.

Not Choosing the Right Type Of IF

Intermittent Fasting doesn't refer to a single method; there are several. One is the 5:2 fast, where a person consumes a normal number of calories for five days and restricts their diet to less than half that number of calories for two days.

Then there is 24-hour IF, time-restrictive IF (where you eat only between four and five hours a day and fast for the rest of the day), and alternate-day IF. Choose the one that fits your goals, schedule, and comfort level.

Too Fast, Too Soon

When you practice Intermittent Fasting, you distance yourself from your usual way of living and eating. This puts some stress on your mental and physical health. Then there's the risk of procrastination and quitting too soon.

If you're a woman who snacks every two hours, then putting yourself into a hard-core straight 16 or 20-hour fasting routine might not turn out well. But your chances of success with IF will increase if you start with seven to eight hours of fasting.

Over-Stretching Fasting Time

The importance of starting low is also important to pace your fasting period. For example, if you've started fasting for eight hours, your next milestone should be as near the 8 hours as possible. So, 10 or 12 hours is a better milestone than 15 hours.

Not Adjusting with Lifestyle

Intermittent Fasting is like a ritual, and there are many factors in your everyday life that can influence it, one of them is the lifestyle you lead. You will set yourself up for misery if you deliberately sign up for that something you know will clash with your fasting activity.

For example, if you're a gym-goer and train heavily for two to three hours, then if you follow it up with a 16 hour fast, it's prone to give health complications. Similarly, if you're going out or have birthday plans during the week, you should plan your IF to avoid clashing with these plans.

Eliminating Exercise Completely

While fasting, it's imperative to think that exercising is useless since you're not eating anything, and the body is not getting the energy it needs to help you do your workout. But an average person has enough energy stored in the body to get you through your workout routine without feeling exhausted.

While you can't perform your usual drill session, you can do low-impact exercises like walking, cycling, or jogging. It will keep your body's metabolism going, taking you faster towards your goals.

For example, if you're planning to fast overnight, then you can hit the gym in the morning and have your protein shakes to build up muscles.

Not Listening to Your Body

It's a fact that we all are different biologically. So, we cannot have one single rule that is meant to follow by everyone on this planet. The online information about Intermittent Fasting is very general. To get the most out of your Intermittent Fasting, you tailor it to your requirements.

For example, your stomach might start acting up after fasting for 4 to 5 hours. Now, as a rule of IF, you cannot eat anything during the fasting window. But if you continue following this rule, then chances are you'll develop some medical complications.

Therefore, you'd require an IF plan specific to your body. If you're having some problems when you're fasting, it's best to consult with a doctor.

Not Persisting With It

Finally, women who start Intermittent Fasting give up too soon or after a few months, stating that it's not for them, it doesn't work, or they simply cannot do it. Barring any medical complications, you must push yourself through the fasting hours and stick with it to realize the amazing benefits of this technique. You've to give it at least one and a half to two months to see some significant results.

CHAPTER 10

1. Swiss and Pear Omelet

Preparation Time: **10 minutes**

Cooking Time: **10 minutes**

Servings: **1**

Ingredients:

- 1 1/2 oz. Shredded Swiss cheese

- 1 1/2 tbsp. Almond milk

- 3 pcs. Eggs

- 1/4 tsp.Salt

- 1/4 pc. Chopped pear

- 1 pc. Diced shallot

- 1 tbsp. Olive oil

Directions:

1. Heat a skillet. While it's heating up, cut up a pear into thin slices. When the skillet is warm, add the salt, sliced pear, and shallot and cook for 5 minutes.

2. While that is cooking, using a bowl, whisk together the almond milk and eggs. Pour into the same skillet at the pear mixture.

3. Once you see that the edges are turning white and that the bottom has started to cook, flip your omelet over.

4. Add the cheese to the middle and fold the omelet in half. Cook until the cheese is melted.

Nutrition:

Calories: 121, Carbs: 8 g, Fat: 12 g, Protein: 14 g

2. Breakfast Quesadillas

Preparation Time: **10 minutes**

Cooking Time: **15 minutes**

Servings: **1**

Ingredients:

- 1 pc. Chopped green onion
- 1 pc. Egg
- 1 pc. Tortilla
- Salt
- Chili powder
- 1/2 tbsp. Water
- 1/2 tbsp. Chunky salsa
- 1/2 tbsp. Refried beans
- 2 tbsp. Cheddar cheese

Directions:

1. Whisk the water and the egg together with the chili powder.

2. Place a skillet on the stove and heat it. Then, cook the green onion until it is tender before reducing the heat to a medium setting.

3. Pour your egg mixture into the skillet and continue stirring until it is the desired consistency. Turn the heat off and cover this up to keep it warm.

4. On a clean counter, spread the tortilla out and add the salsa and beans. Add the egg on top of this and then top with cheese.

5. Wipe the skillet clean and place it on a low flame. Heat the pan, then add the quesadilla, and cook for a few minutes on each side.

6. Move the dish to a plate and keep warm before serving.

Calories: 190, Carbs: 25 g, Fat: 11 g, Protein: 8 g

3. Ham and Asparagus Casserole

Preparation Time: **15 minutes**

Cooking Time: **20 minutes**

Servings: **1**

Ingredients:

- 1/2 Cheddar cheese
- 1/2 Cooked ham
- 1/2 Flour
- 1 cup Nonfat milk
- 2 pcs. Chopped asparagus
- 4 pcs. Eggs
- 1 pc. Chopped red bell pepper
- 1 pc. Chopped onion
- Pepper
- Salt
- 1/4 tsp. Tarragon
- 2 tbsp. Parmesan

Directions:

1. Preheat the oven to 425 degrees.

2. Grease a baking dish with cooking spray. Spread out the ham on the bottom, followed by the bell pepper, onion, and asparagus.

3. Using a bowl, whisk together the salt, pepper, dried tarragon, milk, flour, Parmesan cheese, and eggs. Mix well.

4. Pour the egg mixture over the other ingredients in your baking dish. Place the baking dish in the oven and let it bake.

5. Cook for 10 minutes or until the casserole is set, then you can take it out of the oven. Add the cheddar cheese and then bake for another 2 minutes or until cheese is melted.

6. Allow it to stand on the cooling rack for a few minutes before serving.

Nutrition:

Calories: 190, Carbs: 5 g, Fat: 11 g, Protein: 12 g

4. Blueberry Compote and Yogurt

Preparation Time: **5 minutes**

Cooking Time: **3 minutes**

Servings: **1**

Ingredients:

- 1 tsp. Bran

- 3 tbsp. Fat-free yogurt

- 50 pcs. Blueberries

Directions:

1. Place the blueberries inside a bowl. Then, put them in the microwave on the high setting for about 45 seconds so that the blueberries will start to burst.

2. Take the bowl out of the microwave and let it cool down.

3. When the blueberries are cooked, top with the bran and the yogurt before serving.

Nutrition:

Calories: 75, Carbs: 11 g, Fat: 5 g, Protein: 1 g

5. Sweet Potato Pancakes

Preparation Time: **10 minutes**

Cooking Time: **50 minutes**

Servings: **3**

Ingredients:

- 1 1/2 tbsp. Maple syrup
- 1/4 tsp. Nutmeg
- 1 tsp. Cinnamon
- 4 Egg whites
- 5 Eggs
- 1 1/2 Oats
- 1 1/2 Cottage cheese
- 2 pcs. Sweet potatoes

Directions:

1. Preheat the oven to 400 degrees.

2. Put the potatoes and prick them a few times with a fork. Add them to a baking sheet and let them cook about 50 minutes until they are softened.

3. Take the sweet potatoes out of the oven and carefully slit them lengthwise. Allow these to cool before separating the potato from the skin. Place the potatoes in the blender.

4. Add the syrup, nutmeg, cinnamon, egg whites, eggs, oats, and cottage cheese into the blender. Blend this until you reach a smooth consistency.

5. Prepare a big skillet with cooking spray and place it on medium heat. When hot, scoop some of the batter onto the skillet and cook until the pancakes become golden brown, which will take about 4 minutes.

6. Repeat with the rest and then serve warm.

Nutrition:

Calories: 238, Carbs: 28 g, Fat: 6 g, Protein: 18 g

6. Blueberry Scones

Preparation Time: 15 minutes

Cooking Time: 15 minutes

Servings: 6

Ingredients:

- 1/2 tsp. Salt

- 4 tsp. Baking powder

- 1/8 cup Whole-wheat flour

- 1 1/4 Flour

- Cooking spray

- 1 cup Wild blueberries

- 1 tsp. Vanilla

- 1/2 cup Milk

- 1 cup Greek yogurt

- 3 tbsp. Canola oil

- 1 pc. Egg

- 1/2 Sugar

- 1/4 Baking soda

Directions:

1. Preheat the oven to 400 degrees. Take out two baking sheets and coat with cooking spray.

2. In a bowl, sift both types of flour with the baking soda, salt, and baking powder.

3. In a second bowl, add the vanilla, milk, yogurt, oil, egg, and sugar. Fold the dry ingredients in with the wet ingredients until mixed. Add the blueberries last and continue to mix well.

4. Place a generous spoonful of the batter onto the baking sheets, leaving space between each scone. Place the baking pans into the oven for 15 minutes.

5. Remove the scones from the oven and let them cool before serving.

Nutrition:

Calories: 160, Carbs: 26 g, Fat: 4 g, Protein: 5 g

7. Mini Quiche

Preparation Time: 15 minutes

Cooking Time: 30 minutes

Servings: 6

Ingredients:

- 2 tsp. Olive oil
- 1/4 tsp. Pepper
- 1/2 tsp. Salt
- 1 tbsp. Rosemary
- 1/8 Parmesan cheese
- 6 pcs. Egg whites
- 5 pcs. Eggs
- Cooking spray
- 3 oz. Baby spinach
- 6 oz. Mushrooms
- 1 pc. Minced garlic cloves
- 1/2 cup Chopped red onion

Directions:

1. Preheat the oven to 350 degrees. Coat some muffin tins with cooking spray and add liners to each one.

2. In a bowl, whisk together the pepper, salt, rosemary, Parmesan cheese, egg whites, and eggs to make them fluffy.

3. Take out a skillet and heat the olive oil. Add the garlic and onion, then cook for a couple of minutes to release their aroma.

4. Put the mushrooms and cook for another 5 minutes.

5. Take the pan off the heat and let it cool down a little bit. Place some of this mixture into each of the prepared muffin cups and add some spinach on the top.

6. Slowly pour the egg mixture into each cup and fill them to the rim. Add these to the oven and let them bake.

7. After 25 minutes, take them out of the oven and allow them to cool down before serving.

Nutrition:

Calories: 83, Carbs: 2 g, Fat: 5 g, Protein: 8 g

8. Apple Walnut Loaf

Preparation Time: **20 minutes**

Cooking Time: **55 minutes**

Servings: **1**

Ingredients:

- ½ cup Apple sauce
- 1/2 tsp. Cinnamon
- 1/2 tsp. Salt
- 1 tsp. Baking soda
- 1 cup All-purpose flour
- 1 cup Whole-wheat flour
- Cooking spray
- 1/2 cup Chopped walnuts
- 1 pc. Chopped Rome apple
- 1/2 cupUnsweetened almond milk
- 1 pc. Egg
- 1/2 cup Honey

Directions:

1. Preheat the oven to 325 degrees.

2. Prepare a loaf pan and put some cooking spray.

3. Take out a medium bowl and sift together the all-purpose and whole-wheat flours with the cinnamon, salt, and baking soda.

4. In another bowl, combine the honey and applesauce. Then, add the almond milk and egg and stir well.

5. Fold the dry ingredients into this, but be careful not to overmix. Fold in the walnuts and the apples in as well, making sure to distribute them evenly throughout the batter.

6. Pour this batter into a loaf pan and spread it out evenly. Add this to the oven and allow to bake for 55 minutes.

7. Cool for at 5 minutes before cutting into slices.

Nutrition:

Calories: 206, Carbs: 45 g, Fat: 2 g, Protein: 5 g

9. Cherry and Almond Breakfast Cookies

Preparation Time: **20 minutes**

Cooking Time: **15 minutes**

Servings: **6**

Ingredients:

- 1 tsp. Baking soda
- 2 cups Whole-wheat flour
- 1/2 cup Rolled oats
- Cooking spray
- 1 cup Sliced raw almonds
- 1 cup Chopped tart cherries, dried
- 1 tsp. Vanilla
- 2 pcs. Eggs
- 1/2 cup Maple syrup
- 1/2 cup Brown sugar
- 1/2 cup Plain Greek yogurt
- 1/2 cup Applesauce
- 1/4 tsp. Salt

Directions:

1. Preheat the oven to 350 degrees. Take out a few baking sheets and line them with parchment paper.

2. Using a bowl, and combine the salt, baking soda, flour, and oats.

3. In a second bowl, whisk together the Greek yogurt and applesauce. Mix well, then add in the maple syrup and brown sugar and continue to mix.

4. Add the vanilla and the eggs and mix the ingredients until reaching a smooth, even consistency.

5. Slowly fold the dry ingredients into the wet ones and stir to combine. Add the almonds and cherries, making sure that they are well distributed in the batter.

6. Add 2 tablespoons of batter onto a baking sheet to make each cookie and then flatten them down slightly. Place in the oven to bake.

7. After 15 minutes, you can take the cookies out and let them cool before serving or storing.

8.

Nutrition:

Calories: 214, Carbs: 36 g, Fat: 6 g, Protein: 6 g

10. Peanut Butter Energy Cookies

Preparation Time: **20 minutes**

Cooking Time: **45 minutes**

Servings: **6**

Ingredients:

- 1/2 cup Peanut butter, creamy

- 1/4 tsp. Salt

- 1 tsp. Baking soda

- 1/4 cup Cocoa powder

- 1 cup Flour

- 1/2 cup Chopped peanuts

- 2 cups Rolled oats

- 1 tsp. Vanilla

- 2 pcs. Beaten eggs

- 1/2 cup Brown sugar

- 1/2 cup Milk

- 1/4 cup Greek yogurt

- 1 cup Mashed banana

Directions:

1. Using a bowl, sift together the salt, baking soda, cocoa powder, and flour.

2. In another bowl, mix the milk, Greek yogurt, banana, and peanut butter. Add the brown sugar and then stir to combine.

Finally, add the vanilla and the eggs and combine.

3. Add the flour to the peanut butter mixture along with the oats and peanuts. Stir well until a uniform moist consistency is reached.

4. Place the bowl with cover in the fridge for 30 minutes.

5. Preheat the oven to 350 degrees.

6. Prepare two baking sheets and coat them with cooking spray.

7. Place a spoonful of the batter onto the baking sheet for each cookie, making sure to leave plenty of space between each. You should be able to fit around twelve cookies per sheet.

8. Use a fork to press them down a little bit, giving the cookies the usual crisscross pattern. Place in the oven to bake.

9. Take out the cookies after 15 minutes and allow them to cool down before serving.

Nutrition:

Calories: 143, Carbs: 19 g, Fat: 1 g, Protein: 5 g

CHAPTER 11

1. Mushrooms and Sausage Gravy

Preparation Time: **10 minutes**

Cooking Time: **15 minutes**

Servings: **1**

Ingredients:

- 1-pound Italian ground sausage

- 2 Tablespoons coconut oil

- 1 yellow onion, diced

- 2 garlic cloves, minced

- 2 cups mushrooms, chopped

- 1 red bell pepper, minced

- 2 Tablespoons ghee, melted

- 1/3 cup coconut flour

- 3 1/2 cups coconut milk, unsweetened

- 1/2 cup organic heavy cream

- 1 teaspoon salt (to taste)

- 1 tsp. ground black pepper (to taste)

1. Press the Sauté button on Instant Pot. Heat the coconut oil. Sauté onion and garlic for 2 minutes.

2. Add the Italian sausage. Cook until brown.

3. Add mushrooms, bell peppers and sauté until soft. Season with salt and pepper.

4. Press the Keep Warm/Cancel button to end Sauté mode.

5. In a small saucepan, over medium heat, melt the ghee. Add the flour. Whisk in coconut milk and heavy cream. Continue stirring until thickens.

6. Add flour mixture to Instant Pot. Stir well.

7. Close and seal lid. Press the Manual button. Cook at High Pressure for 10 minutes.

8. When the timer beeps, naturally release pressure. Open the lid with care. Serve.

Nutrition:

Calories: 115, Fat: 7 g, Carbs: 9 g, Protein: 5 g

2. Asparagus and Shrimp Mix

Preparation Time: **10 minutes**

Cooking Time: **6 minutes**

Servings: **1**

Ingredients:

- 1 pound asparagus, trimmed and chopped
- 1 pound shrimp, peeled and deveined
- 2 tablespoons ghee, melted
- 2 cups of water
- 1 teaspoon salt (to taste)
- 1 tsp. ground black pepper (to taste)

Directions:

1. Put 2 cups of water in Instant Pot.

2. Place shrimp and asparagus in a steamer basket. Drizzle melted ghee over shrimp and asparagus. Season with salt and pepper. Place basket in Instant Pot.

3. Close and seal lid. Press the Manual button. Cook at High Pressure for 6 minutes.

4. When the timer beeps, release pressure naturally. Open the lid with care. Serve.

Nutrition:

Calories: 155, Fat: 1 g, Carbs: 15 g, Protein: 23 g

3. Collard Greens and Bacon

Preparation Time: **10 minutes**

Cooking Time: **15 minutes**

Servings: **1**

Ingredients:

- 1 pound collard greens, trimmed and chopped
- ¼ pound bacon, chopped
- ½ cup ghee, melted
- 1 teaspoon salt
- 1 teaspoon fresh ground black pepper

Directions:

1. Press the Sauté button on Instant Pot. Melt 1 tablespoon of ghee. Add the bacon. Sauté until bacon is brown and crispy. Press the Keep Warm/Cancel button to end Sauté mode.

2. Add collard greens, the rest of the ghee, salt and pepper. Stir well.

3. Close and seal lid. Press the Manual button. Cook at High Pressure for 10 minutes.

4. When done, naturally release pressure. Open the lid with care. Stir. Serve.

Nutrition:

Calories: 125, Fat: 9 g, Carbs: 4 g, Protein: 7 g

4. Spaghetti Squash

Preparation Time: **5 minutes**

Cooking Time: **7 minutes**

Servings: **2**

Ingredients:

- 1 (2 pounds) spaghetti squash, cut half lengthwise
- 1 cup of water

Directions:

1. Add 1 cup of water and a steamer basket or trivet inside your Instant Pot.
2. Place the squash on top. Lock the lid and cook at high pressure for 7 minutes.
3. When the cooking is done, manually release the pressure and remove the lid.
4. Shred the spaghetti squash using two forks.
5. Serve and enjoy.

Nutrition:

Calories: 45, Fat: 0.4 g, Carbs: 10 g, Protein: 1 g

5. Ultimate Corn on the Cob

Preparation Time: **5 minutes**

Cooking Time: **5 minutes**

Servings: **8**

Ingredients:

- 8 corn on the cob
- 2 cups of water
- 2 teaspoons low-carb brown sugar
- 1 teaspoon salt (to taste)
- 1 tsp. ground black pepper (to taste)

Directions:

1. Place corn in a steamer basket with 2 cups of water. Place basket in Instant Pot.
2. Close and seal lid. Press the Manual button. Cook at High Pressure for 5 minutes.
3. When the timer beeps, naturally release pressure. Open the lid with care.
4. Sprinkle with brown sugar.
5. Serve.

Nutrition:

Calories: 99, Fat: 1 g, Carbs: 22 g, Protein: 3 g

6. Chicken and Broccoli Casserole

Preparation Time: **10 minutes**

Cooking Time: **50 minutes**

Servings: **1**

Ingredients:

- 1 pound of broccoli florets
- 3 boneless, skinless chicken breasts, cut into bite-sized pieces
- 3 cups of cheddar cheese, shredded or finely grated
- 1 cup of homemade zero-sugar mayonnaise
- 2 tablespoons of coconut oil, melted
- ½ teaspoon of freshly cracked black pepper
- 1/3 cup of homemade low-sodium chicken stock
- ½ teaspoon of sea salt
- 2 tablespoons of freshly squeezed lemon juice

Directions:

1. Preheat your oven to 350 degrees Fahrenheit. Grease a baking dish with the coconut oil.

2. Place the chicken pieces to the bottom of the baking dish.

3. Spread the broccoli florets on top of the chicken.

4. Spread half of the shredded cheddar cheese over the broccoli.

5. In a bowl, add the mayonnaise, chicken stock, sea salt, freshly cracked black pepper, and lemon juice. Pour this mixture over the chicken.

6. Sprinkle the remaining cheddar cheese over the baking dish and tightly cover the aluminum foil.

7. Place the baking dish inside your oven and bake for 30 minutes.

8. Once done, remove the baking dish from your oven and carefully remove the aluminum foil. Return the baking dish to your oven and bake for 20 minutes.

9. Serve and enjoy.

Nutrition:

Calories: 280, Fat: 7 g, Carbs: 16 g, Protein: 37 g

7. Italian-Inspired Chicken Breast

Preparation Time: **15 minutes**

Cooking Time: **15 minutes**

Servings: **4**

Ingredients:

- 4 boneless, skinless chicken breasts
- 1 pound of cherry tomatoes, halved
- 4 garlic cloves, finely minced
- ¼ cup of olive oil or extra-virgin olive oil
- 1 medium red onion, finely chopped
- ½ cup of green olives, pitted and chopped
- 4 anchovy fillets, chopped
- 1 tablespoon of capers, chopped
- 1 teaspoon of sea salt
- 1 teaspoon of freshly cracked black pepper

Directions:

1. Preheat your oven to 450 degrees Fahrenheit.
2. Mix the chicken breast with sea salt and black pepper. Rub half of the olive oil with the chicken breasts.
3. Place a skillet over high heat. Add the chicken breast and cook for 2 minutes per side.
4. Transfer the chicken breasts to a baking pan.
5. Transfer the chicken breasts to a baking pan. Place the baking

pan inside your oven and bake for 8 minutes.

6. Once done, transfer the chicken breasts on plates. Set aside.

7. Add the chopped onion, minced garlic, chopped olives, anchovies, halved cherry tomatoes and capers to the skillet. Cook for 1 minute, stirring occasionally.

8. Drizzle the tomato mixture over the chicken breasts.

9. Transfer to containers and enjoy.

Nutrition:

Calories: 190, Fat: 11 g, Carbs: 1 g, Protein: 19 g

8. Lemon Chicken

Preparation Time: 15 minutes

Cooking Time: 45 minutes

Servings: 6

Ingredients:

- 6 boneless, skinless chicken breasts or chicken thighs

- 1 medium onion, chopped

- 6 garlic cloves, minced

- 2 tablespoons of olive oil

- 2 teaspoons of sea salt

- 2 teaspoons of freshly cracked black pepper

- Juice and zest from 2 medium-sized lemons

- 1 lemon, cut into wedges

Directions:

1. Preheat your oven to 375 degrees Fahrenheit.

2. Prepare a baking dish and put the chicken. Season with sea salt and black pepper.

3. Add the chopped onion, minced garlic, lemon juice, olive oil and lemon zest. Stir until well incorporated.

4. Add the lemon wedges.

5. Place the baking dish inside your oven and bake for 45 minutes or until the chicken is cooked through.

6. Get the baking dish from your oven and discard the lemon wedges.

7. Transfer the lemon chicken to containers and enjoy.

Nutrition:

Calories: 280, Fat: 5 g, Carbs: 1 g, Protein: 55 g

9. Hearty Lemon & Garlic Pork

Preparation Time: **10 minutes**

Cooking Time: **20 minutes**

Servings: **4**

Ingredients:

- 4 pork chops, boneless
- 2 cups beef broth
- 3 tablespoons ghee, melted
- 3 tablespoons coconut oil
- 1 teaspoon salt
- 1 teaspoon fresh ground black pepper
- Zest and juice from 2 lemons
- 6 garlic cloves, minced
- ¼ cup fresh parsley, chopped

Directions:

1. Mix the pork chops with salt and pepper, lemon juice and zest.
2. Press the Sauté button on your Instant Pot. Heat coconut oil.
3. Sauté garlic for 1 minute. Add pork chops. Sear for 2 minutes per side.
4. Press the Keep Warm/Cancel button to end Sauté mode.
5. Add ghee and beef broth to the Instant Pot. Close and seal lid. Press the Poultry button. Cook for 15 minutes.

6. Quick-release pressure when done. Open the lid with care. Stir ingredients.

7. Serve.

Nutrition:

Calories: 158, Fat: 6 g, Carbs: 7 g, Protein: 20 g

10. Tasty Thai Beef

Preparation Time: **15 minutes**

Cooking Time: **25 minutes**

Servings: **1**

Ingredients:

- 1 pound of beef, cut into strips
- 1 green bell pepper, chopped
- 1 red bell pepper, chopped
- Zest and juice from 1 lemon
- 2 cups beef broth
- 2 teaspoons ginger, grated
- 4 garlic cloves, minced
- 2 tablespoons coconut oil
- 1 tablespoon coconut amino
- 1 cup roasted pecans
- 1 teaspoon salt
- 1 teaspoon fresh ground black pepper

Directions:

1. Press the Sauté button on Instant Pot. Heat the coconut oil.

2. Sauté garlic and ginger for 1 minute. Add the beef strips. Sear 1-2 minutes per side.

3. Add bell peppers. Add salt and pepper. Cook until meat is no longer pink.

4. Add coconut amino, pecans, zest and juice from lemon, beef broth. Stir well.

5. Close and seal lid. Press Manual setting. Cook at High Pressure for 15 minutes.

6. Release pressure naturally when done. Open the lid with care. Let it sit for 5 – 10 minutes.

Nutrition:

Calories: 200, Fat: 6 g, Carbs: 17 g, Protein: 23 g

11. Gratifying Meatloaf

Preparation Time: **20 minutes**

Cooking Time: **30 minutes**

Servings: **1**

Ingredients:

- 3 pounds lean ground beef
- 4 garlic cloves, minced
- 1 yellow onion, chopped
- 1 cup mushrooms, chopped
- 3 large eggs
- ½ cup almond flour
- ¼ cup parmesan cheese, grated
- ¼ cup mozzarella cheese, grated
- ¼ cup fresh parsley, chopped
- 2 tablespoons sugar-free ketchup
- 2 tablespoons coconut oil
- 2 teaspoons salt
- 2 teaspoons black pepper
- 2 cups of water

Directions:

1. Cover trivet with aluminum foil.

2. Mix all the ingredients excluding, the water in a large bowl until well combined.

3. Form into a meatloaf. Pour the water in your Instant Pot.

4. Place meatloaf on the trivet.

5. Close and seal lid. Press the Manual button. Cook at High-Pressure for 25 minutes.

6. Release pressure naturally when done. Open the lid with care.

7. Rest the meatloaf for 5 minutes before slicing and serve.

Nutrition:

Calories: 163, Fat: 3 g, Carbs: 21 g, Protein: 19 g

12. Herbed Salmon Fillets

Preparation Time: **15 minutes**

Cooking Time: **10 minutes**

Servings: **4**

Ingredients:

- 4 (6-ounce) boneless salmon fillets
- 1 tablespoon of fresh parsley, chopped
- 1 tablespoon of fresh basil, chopped
- 1 tablespoon of fresh thyme, chopped
- 4 fresh rosemary sprigs
- 4 whole garlic cloves
- ½ teaspoon of freshly cracked black pepper
- 2 tablespoons of olive oil
- ½ teaspoon of sea salt
- ½ teaspoon of onion powder
- 2 lemons, sliced

Directions:

1. Preheat your oven to 390 degrees Fahrenheit.

2. In a bowl, add the fresh parsley, fresh basil, fresh thyme, olive oil, sea salt, black pepper, and onion powder. Mix until well combined.

3. Grease a baking sheet and place the salmon fillets on top.

4. Add the herbed mixture over the salmon and gently place lemon slices, rosemary sprig, and whole garlic cloves.

5. Place inside your oven and bake for 10 to 13 minutes or until cooked through.

6. Serve and enjoy.

Nutrition:

Calories: 220, Fat: 13 g, Carbs: 4 g, Protein: 22 g

CHAPTER 12

DINNER RECIPES

1. Aromatic Zucchini Noodles Soup

Preparation Time: **25 minutes**

Cooking Time: **15 minutes**

Servings: **2**

Ingredients:

- 1pound chicken breasts; sliced
- 6 cups chicken stock
- 15 ounces canned coconut milk
- 1 red bell pepper; sliced
- 1 tablespoon coconut oil
- 1½ tablespoons curry paste
- 2 zucchinis; cut with a spiralizer
- 2 tablespoons fish sauce
- 1 small yellow onion; chopped.
- 2 garlic cloves; minced
- 1 jalapeno pepper; chopped.

- 1/2 cup cilantro; chopped.
- Lime wedges for serving

1. Heat a pot with the oil over medium heat; add onion; stir and cook for 5 minutes
2. Add garlic, jalapeno and curry paste; stir and cook for 1 minute.
3. Add stock and coconut milk; stir and bring to a boil.
4. Add red bell pepper, chicken and fish sauce; stir and simmer for 4 minutes more.
5. Add cilantro; stir, cook for 1 minute and take off the heat.
6. Divide zucchini noodles into soup bowls, add soup on top and serve with lime wedges on the side.

Nutrition:

Calories: 250, Fat: 5 g, Carbs: 21 g, Protein: 34 g

2. Pizza

Preparation Time: **20 minutes**

Cooking Time: **30 minutes**

Servings: **2**

Ingredients:

- 1 cup pizza cheese mix; shredded
- 1 tablespoon olive oil
- 2 tablespoons ghee
- 1 cup mozzarella cheese; shredded
- 1/3 cup broccoli florets; steamed
- 1/4 cup mascarpone cheese
- Some asiago cheese; shaved for serving
- 1 teaspoon garlic; minced
- 1 tablespoon heavy cream
- A pinch of lemon pepper
- Salt and black pepper to the taste.

Directions:

1. Heat a pan with the oil over medium heat.
2. Add pizza cheese mix and spread into a circle.
3. Add mozzarella cheese and also spread into a circle.
4. Cook everything for 5 minutes and transfer to a plate.
5. Heat the pan with the ghee over medium heat; add mascarpone cheese, cream, salt, pepper, lemon pepper and garlic; stir and

cook for 5 minutes.

6. Drizzle half of this mix over cheese crust.

7. Add broccoli florets to the pan with the rest of the mascarpone mix; stir and cook for 1 minute.

8. Add this on top of the pizza, sprinkle asiago cheese at the end and serve.

Nutrition:

Calories: 304, Fat: 7 g, Carbs: 50 g, Protein: 9 g

3. Lobster Bisque

Preparation Time: **25 minutes**

Cooking Time: **1 hour and 10 minutes**

Servings: **2**

Ingredients:

- 24 ounces lobster chunks, pre-cooked
- 1/2 cup tomato paste
- 4 garlic cloves, minced
- 1 small red onion, chopped.
- 1 teaspoon thyme, dried
- 1 teaspoon peppercorns
- 1 teaspoon paprika
- 1 teaspoon xanthan gum
- 2 carrots finely chopped.
- 4 celery stalks, chopped.
- 1 quart seafood stock
- 1 tablespoon olive oil
- 1 cup heavy cream
- 3 bay leaves
- A handful parsley, chopped.
- 1 tablespoon lemon juice
- Salt and black pepper to the taste.

1. Heat a pot with the oil over medium heat.

2. Add onion and cook for 4 minutes.

3. Put garlic, celery and carrot and cook for 1 minute more.

4. Add the tomato paste and stock. Stir.

5. Put bay leaves, salt, pepper, peppercorns, paprika, thyme and xanthan gum then simmer over medium heat for 1 hour.

6. Remove bay leaves and add cream then bring to a simmer.

7. Blend using an immersion blender, add lobster chunks and cook for a few minutes more

8. Add lemon juice; stir, divide into bowls and sprinkle parsley on top.

Nutrition:

Calories: 370, Fat: 31 g, Carbs: 16 g, Protein: 7 g

4. Pumpkin Soup

Preparation Time: **15 minutes**

Cooking Time: **15 minutes**

Servings: **3**

Ingredients:

- 2 cups pumpkin puree
- 1/2 cup heavy cream
- 1/2 cup yellow onion; chopped.
- 32 ounces chicken stock
- 1 garlic clove; minced
- 1 teaspoon cumin; ground
- 1 teaspoon coriander; ground
- 2 teaspoons vinegar
- 2 teaspoons stevia
- 2 tablespoons olive oil
- 1 tablespoon chipotles in adobo sauce
- A pinch of allspice
- Salt and black pepper to the taste.

Directions:

1. Heat a pot with the oil over medium heat; add onions and garlic; stir and cook for 4 minutes
2. Add stevia, cumin, coriander, chipotles and cumin; stir and cook for 2 minutes

3. Add stock and pumpkin puree; stir and cook for 5 minutes

4. Blend soup well using an immersion blender and then mix with salt, pepper, heavy cream and vinegar.

5. Stir, cook for 5 minutes more and divide into bowls Serve right away.

Nutrition:

Calories: 115, Fat: 4 g, Carbs: 16 g, Protein: 3 g

5. Juicy Brussels Sprouts

Preparation Time: **15 minutes**

Cooking Time: **10 minutes**

Servings: **4**

Ingredients:

- 1lb. Brussels sprouts; trimmed
- 1/4 cup green onions; chopped.
- 6 cherry tomatoes; halved
- 1 tablespoon olive oil
- Salt and black pepper to the taste

Directions:

1. Toss brussels sprouts with salt and black pepper in a baking dish.

2. Cook the sprouts for 10minutes at 350 degrees F in a preheated oven.

3. Toss these sprouts with green onions, tomatoes, olive oil, salt and pepper in a salad bowl.

4. Devour.

Nutrition:

Calories 135, Fat 10 g, Carbs 11 g, Protein 4 g

6. Baked Cheese Asparagus

Preparation Time: **10 minutes**

Cooking Time: **8 minutes**

Servings: **4**

Ingredients:

- 2 lb. fresh asparagus; trimmed
- 1/2 teaspoon oregano; dried
- 4 oz. feta cheese; crumbled
- 4 garlic cloves; minced
- 1/4 cup olive oil
- Salt and black pepper to the taste

Directions:

1. Toss asparagus, with salt, oregano, garlic, oil, pepper, and cheese in a bowl.

2. Cook them for 8 minutes at 350 degrees F in a preheated oven.

3. Enjoy warm.

Nutrition:

Calories 309, Fat 23 g, Carbs 5 g, Protein 22 g

7. Tofu Pesto Peppers

Preparation Time: **10 minutes**

Cooking Time: **15 minutes**

Servings: **4**

Ingredients:

- 12 baby bell peppers; cut into halves lengthwise
- 1 lb. tofu, diced
- 6 tablespoon jarred basil pesto
- 1 tablespoon olive oil
- 1/4 teaspoon red pepper flakes; crushed
- Salt and black pepper to the taste

Directions:

1. Spread the tofu in a baking sheet and bake for 7 minutes at 350 degrees.
2. Toss tofu with pesto, salt, black pepper, pepper flakes, and oil in a bowl.
3. Stuff the bell peppers with the tofu mixture and place them in a baking sheet.
4. Cook them for 6 minutes at 320 degrees F in the preheated oven.
5. Enjoy.

Nutrition:

Calories 349, Fat 14 g, Carbs 26 g, Protein 30 g

8. Parmesan Tomatoes

Preparation Time: **10 minutes**

Cooking Time: **15 minutes**

Servings: **4**

Ingredients:

- 1 jalapeno pepper; chopped
- 4 garlic cloves; minced
- 1/4 cup olive oil
- 1/2 cup parmesan; grated
- 2 lb. cherry tomatoes; halved
- Salt and black pepper to the taste

Directions:

1. Toss tomatoes with salt, garlic, jalapeno, black pepper and olive oil in a baking dish.
2. Cook the tomatoes for 15 minutes at 380 degrees in a preheated oven.
3. Garnish with parmesan.
4. Enjoy.

Nutrition:

Calories 180, Total Fat 5 g, Total Carbs 32 g, Protein 1 g

9. Tomato Kebabs

Preparation Time: **15 minutes**

Cooking Time: **10 minutes**

Servings: **6**

Ingredients:

- 3 tablespoon balsamic vinegar
- 24 cherry tomatoes
- 2 tablespoon olive oil
- 3 garlic cloves; minced
- 1 tablespoon thyme; chopped
- Salt and black pepper to the taste

Directions:

1. Take a medium bowl and add 1 tablespoon oil, 3 garlic cloves, thyme, salt, and black pepper.
2. Mix well then toss in the tomatoes and coat them liberally.
3. Thread 6 tomatoes on each skewer.
4. Grill the tomato skewers for 3 minutes per side in a preheated grill.
5. Meanwhile, whisk pepper, salt, and 1 tablespoon oil.
6. Place the cooked skewers on the serving plates.
7. Pour the vinegar dressing over them.
8. Enjoy.

Nutrition:

Calories 45, Carbs 9 g, Protein 1 g

10. Garlic Broccoli

Preparation Time: **10 minutes**

Cooking Time: **10 minutes**

Servings: **2**

Ingredients:

- 1 broccoli head; florets separated
- 6 garlic cloves; minced
- 1 tablespoon Chinese rice wine vinegar
- 1 tablespoon peanut oil
- Salt and black pepper to the taste

Directions:

1. Toss broccoli with salt, half of the oil and black pepper in a large bowl.
2. Spread the broccoli in a baking sheet and bake for 8 minutes at 350-degrees F.
3. Mix the cooked broccoli with garlic, peanut oil and rice vinegar in a salad bowl.
4. Serve fresh.

Nutrition:

Calories 170, Fat 11 g, Carbs 11 g, Protein 10 g

11. Halloumi Salad

Preparation Time: **15 minutes**

Cooking Time: **10 minutes**

Servings: **1**

Ingredients:

- 3 ounces halloumi cheese, sliced
- 1 cucumber, sliced
- A handful baby arugula
- 5 cherry tomatoes, halved
- A splash of balsamic vinegar
- 1-ounce walnuts, chopped.
- A drizzle of olive oil
- Salt and black pepper to the taste.

Directions:

1. Heat your kitchen grill over medium-high heat; add halloumi pieces, grill them for 5 minutes on each side and transfer to a plate
2. In a bowl, mix tomatoes with cucumber, walnuts and arugula.
3. Add halloumi pieces on top, season everything with salt, pepper, drizzle the oil and the vinegar, toss to coat and serve

Nutrition:

Calories: 135, Fat: 10 g, Carbs: 7 g, Protein: 3

12. Tomato Soup

Preparation Time: **15 minutes**

Cooking Time: **10 minutes**

Servings: **4**

Ingredients:

- 8 bacon strips, cooked and crumbled
- 4 tablespoons ghee
- 1/4 cup olive oil
- 1/4 cup red hot sauce
- A handful basil leaves, chopped.
- 1-quart canned tomato soup
- 1 teaspoon oregano, dried
- 2 teaspoon turmeric, ground
- A handful green onions, chopped.
- 2 tablespoons apple cider vinegar
- Salt and black pepper to the taste.

Directions:

1. Put tomato soup in a pot and heat up over medium heat.
2. Add olive oil, ghee, hot sauce, vinegar, salt, pepper, turmeric, and oregano; stir and simmer for 5 minutes
3. Take off heat; divide the soup into bowls, top with bacon crumbles, basil and green onions

Nutrition:

Calories: 157, Fat: 1 g, Carbs: 32 g, Protein: 4 g

13. Butter Glazed Carrots

Preparation Time: **10 minutes**

Cooking Time: **10 minutes**

Servings: **4**

Ingredients:

- 2 cups baby carrots
- 1 tablespoon brown swerve
- 1/2 tablespoon butter; melted
- A pinch of salt and black pepper

Directions:

1. Start by tossing carrots with swerve, butter, salt, and black peppers.
2. Spread the glazed carrots in a baking dish.
3. Cook the carrots for 10 minutes at 350 degrees F in a preheated oven.
4. Enjoy.

Nutrition:

Calories 155, Fat 8 g, Carbs 22 g, Protein 1.4 g

14. Tangy Fennel Salad

Preparation Time: **10 minutes**

Cooking Time: **10 minutes**

Servings: **2**

Ingredients:

- 2 fennel bulbs; cut into quarters
- 1 cup veggie stock
- 3 tablespoon olive oil
- Juice from 1/2 lemon
- 1 tablespoon garlic, minced
- Salt and black pepper to the taste

Directions:

1. Start by sautéing garlic with oil in a cooking pan.

2. Add fennel, stock, lemon juice, salt, and pepper.

3. Cook the fennel for 10 minutes on medium-low heat.

4. Serve fresh and warm.

Nutrition:

Calories 98, Fat 9 g, Carbs 3 g, Protein 2 g

15. Spinach Cheese Pie

Preparation Time: **15 minutes**

Cooking Time: **25 minutes**

Servings: **4**

Ingredients:

- 7oz. flour
- 2 tablespoon butter
- 2 eggs
- 2 tablespoon almond milk
- 7oz. spinach
- Salt and black pepper to the taste

Directions:

1. Add flour, butter, salt, pepper, almond milk and 1 egg to a food processor.
2. Blend to get a smooth dough and knead it well.
3. Leave the dough for 10 minutes on the working surface.
4. Whisk egg with spinach, salt, and black pepper.
5. First, divide the dough into four pieces and roll them into ramekin sized crust.
6. Place the crust in the ramekins and press them.
7. Pour the egg mixture in the ramekins.
8. Cook them for 15 minutes approximately at 360 degrees F in a preheated oven.
9. Enjoy warm.

Nutrition:

Calories 160, Fat 2 g, Carbs 6 g, Protein 11 g

CHAPTER 13

1. Sunflower Cookies

Preparation Time: **10 minutes**

Cooking Time: **8 minutes**

Servings: **8**

Ingredients:

- 1 egg
- ½ cup of sunflower seed butter
- 1 tablespoon of coconut oil
- 1 tablespoon of Truvia
- ½ tsp of vanilla extract
- ¼ tsp of baking powder
- ¼ tsp of baking soda
- ¼ tsp of salt

Directions:

1. Set your oven for 360 degrees and get out a slightly greased cookie sheet.

2. While your oven heats, deposit the egg into a mixing bowl, followed by the ½ cup of sunflower seed butter, the tablespoon of coconut oil, the tablespoon of Truvia, the ½ tsp of vanilla extract, the ¼ tsp of baking powder, the ¼ tsp of baking soda, and the ¼ tsp of salt.

3. Stir all of your ingredients together well before using your clean hands to form 8 individual clumps out of the mixture.

4. Arrange your clumps evenly on your greased cooking sheet and place the sheet into the oven.

5. Allow cooking for about 8 minutes or until golden brown.

6. Get the cookies out of the oven and allow to cool.

7. Serve when ready.

Nutrition:

Calories: 70, Protein: 3 g, Carbs: 65 g, Fat: 6 g

2. Homemade Dark Chocolate

Preparation Time: **10 minutes**

Cooking Time: **45 minutes**

Servings: **2**

Ingredients:

- 2 tablespoons of coconut oil
- ¼ cup of cocoa powder
- 2 tablespoons of honey
- 1 tsp of vanilla extract

Directions:

1. Put 2 tablespoons of coconut oil, followed by the ¼ cup of cocoa powder, the 2 tablespoons of honey, and the tsp of vanilla extract to a mixing bowl and spend a few minutes stirring it all together well.

2. Once thoroughly mixed, cover the bowl and place it in the fridge for about 45 minutes.

3. Once chilled and hardened your Homemade Dark Chocolate is ready to eat.

Nutrition:

Calories: 170, Protein: 2 g, Carbs: 15 g, Fat: 3 g

3. Peanut Butter Bars

Preparation Time: **10 minutes**

Cooking Time: **0 minutes**

Servings: **2**

Ingredients:

- 1 cup of peanut butter
- ½ tsp of pure vanilla extract
- ¼ tsp of salt
- 2 tablespoons of almond flour
- ¼ cup of milk

Directions:

1. Put your cup of peanut butter into a mixing bowl, followed by the ½ tsp of pure vanilla extract, the ¼ tsp of salt, the 2 tablespoons of almond flour and the ¼ cup of milk.

2. Stir all of your ingredients together well and pour into an oven safe baking dish.

3. Place the dish in the oven and set temperature for 380 degrees.

4. Cook for about 8 minutes.

5. Take out of the oven and allow cooling at room temperature.

6. Once cool, slice and serve.

Nutrition:

Calories: 116, Protein: 4 g, Carbs: 6 g, Fat: 5 g

4. Low Cal Lemon Curd

Preparation Time: **5 minutes**

Cooking Time: **5 minutes**

Servings: **1-2**

Ingredients:

- ¼ cup of lemon juice

- 1 egg

- ¼ cup of butter

Directions:

1. Prepare a small saucepan, place it onto a burner set for medium heat, and add your ¼ cup of butter.

2. Now add the egg and the ¼ cup of lemon juice and vigorously stir it as it cooks together over the next 5 minutes.

3. Turn the burner off, transfer mixture to a dish and serve.

Nutrition:

Calories: 74, Protein: 1 g, Carbs: 1 g, Fat: 7 g

5. Coconut Avocado Ice Cream

Preparation Time: **5 minutes**

Cooking Time: **4 hours**

Servings: **1**

Ingredients:

- 1 large avocado
- 1 cup of coconut milk
- 1 tablespoon of MCT oil
- 1 tablespoon of lemon juice
- 1 tsp of minced mint leaves
- ¼ tsp of salt

Directions:

1. Remove the skin and pit from your avocado.

2. Put avocado, coconut milk, the tablespoon of MCT oil, the tablespoon of lemon juice, and the teaspoon of minced mint leaves into a blender and blend for about 1 minute.

3. Now pour the mixture into a plastic bowl and place it into your freezer.

4. Freeze for about 4 hours before eating.

5. Serve when ready.

Nutrition:

Calories: 109, Protein: 8 g, Carbs: 11 g, Fat: 90 g

6. Fasting Snickerdoodle Cookies

Preparation Time: **5 minutes**

Cooking Time: **8 minutes**

Servings: **8**

Ingredients:

- 1 cup of butter
- ½ cup of almond flour
- ½ cup of coconut flour
- 1 egg
- ¼ cup of baking powder
- 1 tablespoon of baking soda
- 1 tsp of cinnamon

Directions:

1. Preheat your oven for 350 degrees.

2. Now get out a medium sized mixing bowl and add the cup of butter, followed by the ½ cup of almond flour, the ½ cup of coconut flour, the egg, the ¼ cup of baking powder, the tablespoon of baking soda, and your tsp of cinnamon.

3. Stir all of your mixing bowl ingredients together well before using your (clean) hands to form 8 individual clumps.

4. Arrange your cookie clumps onto a greased baking sheet and place into the oven.

5. Allow cooking for about 8 minutes or until golden brown.

6. Let cookies cool and serve when ready.

Nutrition:

Calories: 105, Protein: 5 g, Carbs: 3 g, Fat: 25 g

7. Chia Seed Pudding

Preparation Time: **10 minutes**

Cooking Time: **3 hours**

Servings: **1-2**

Ingredients:

- ½ cup of coconut milk
- ¼ cup of chia seeds
- 1 tablespoon of Truvia
- 1 tsp of cinnamon
- ¼ tsp of salt

Directions:

7. Take your ½ cup of coconut milk, followed by your ¼ cup of chia seeds, your tablespoon of Truvia, your tsp of cinnamon, your ¼ tsp of salt, and your ¼ tsp of cinnamon and deposit them into a mixing bowl.

8. Stir all of your ingredients together thoroughly for a couple of minutes.

9. Once mixed, place plastic over the bowl and place it in the fridge.

10.   Chill for about 3 hours and serve when ready.

Nutrition:

Calories: 95, Protein: 2 g, Carbs: 2 g, Fat: 10 g

8. Banana Pudding

Preparation Time: **10 minutes**

Cooking Time: **4 hours**

Servings: **1**

Ingredients:

- 1/2 cup heavy cream or ¼ cup heavy and ¼ cup almond milk
- 1 large egg yolk
- 3 tablespoons powdered erythritol
- 1/2 teaspoon xanthan gum
- 1/2 teaspoon banana extract

Directions:

1. Combine the egg yolk, heavy cream (or almond milk and heavy cream), and powdered erythritol.
2. In a double boiler, constantly whisk until the mixture thickens and the erythritol dissolves.
3. Add and whisk the xanthan gum until thickened even more.
4. Add the banana extract and a pinch of salt, stir well.
5. Strain through a sieve, and transfer to the serving dish, cover with a wrap to touch the surface of the pudding.
6. Refrigerate for about 4 hours and enjoy.

Nutrition:

Calories: 130, Fat: 4 g, Carbs: 20 g, Protein: 2 g

9. Strawberry Pistachio Creamsicle

Preparation Time: **10 minutes**

Cooking Time: **2-4 hours**

Servings: **2**

Ingredients:

- 8 oz. strawberries
- 2 oz. salted pistachios
- 1/2 cup heavy cream
- 1/2 cup almond milk
- 2 tsp. stevia

Directions:

1. Place your popsicle molds in the freezer beforehand. This will help accelerate the freezing process.

2. Blend the strawberries, stevia, heavy cream, and almond milk until fully combined. Let this blend for about a minute so the cream has a chance to aerate and whip.

3. Throw your pistachios into the mix and stir, do not blend. You can also use walnuts, cashews, or pecans.

4. Pour the creamsicle mix into your cold popsicle molds and insert the bases. Freeze for about 2 hours or until set.

5. To remove the creamsicle, allow hot water to run against the outside of the popsicle molds. This will melt some of the ice cream that sticks the creamsicle to the molds. Then gently pull on the bases until your ice cream is out.

Nutrition:

Calories: 120, Fat: 6 g, Carbs: 14 g, Protein: 3 g

10. Avocado Chocolate Pudding

Preparation Time: **10 minutes**

Cooking Time: **5 minutes**

Servings: **1**

Ingredients:

- One avocado
- 2 ½ tablespoons raw cocoa powder
- 1/16 teaspoon ground cayenne pepper
- One teaspoon Ceylon cinnamon
- 1 tablespoon coconut milk
- 1 tablespoon erythritol
- 1/2 teaspoon vanilla extract
- 1 pinch stevia
- 1 pinch pink Himalayan sea salt

Directions:

1. Cut and blend the avocado in a food processor.
2. Put cocoa powder, coconut milk, and vanilla extract. Blend until smooth.
3. Add cinnamon, sweetener, ground cayenne pepper, and a bit of stevia.
4. Blend and scrape down the sides of the food processor to get all the chunks.
5. Serve with a sprinkle of coarse Himalayan pink sea salt for a flavorful crunch.

Nutrition:

Calories: 87, Fat: 7 g, Carbs: 9 g, Protein: 1.5

CHAPTER 14

SMOOTHIE RECIPES

1. Pineapple Coconut Deluxe Smoothie

Preparation Time: **5 minutes**

Cooking Time: **5 minutes**

Servings: **2**

Ingredients:

- 1 C pineapple chunks
- 1 C coconut milk
- 1/2 C pineapple juice
- 1 ripe banana
- 1/2 – 3/4 C ice cubes
- Pure liquid stevia to taste
- 1 tablespoon hemp protein powder

Directions:

1. In a blender, combine the pineapple chunks, coconut milk, banana, ice, and pure liquid stevia.

2. Puree until smooth.

3. Pour into two large glasses.

4. Garnish with a pineapple wedge if desired.

Nutrition:

Calories: 120, Carbs: 30 g

2. Divine Vanilla Smoothie

Preparation Time: **5 minutes**

Cooking Time: **5 minutes**

Servings: **2**

Ingredients:

- 1 cup coconut or almond milk
- ¼ cup almond butter
- 1 tsp vanilla paste, (or vanilla extract)
- 2 cups ice
- Sweet Leaf Stevia Vanilla Creme, to taste
- Vanilla hemp Protein Powder – 1 tablespoon

Directions:

1. Add all ingredients except ice to the blender. Puree well.
2. Add ice and blend until ice is all crushed, and smoothie is well blended and smooth.
3. Pour into two glasses and serve immediately.
4. Add more or less ice to make the smoothie thinner or thicker consistency.

Nutrition:

Calories: 130, Fat: 3 g, Carbs: 6 g, Protein: 20 g

3. Coco Orange Delish Smoothie

Preparation Time: **5 minutes**

Cooking Time: **5 minutes**

Servings: **2**

Ingredients:

- 1/2 cup fresh squeezed orange juice
- 1 tablespoon hemp protein powder
- 1/2 cup full fat coconut milk from the can (not the box!)
- 1 teaspoon vanilla
- 1/2 cup crushed ice

Directions:

1. Add all ingredients to a blender.
2. Blend until smooth and add ice as needed to get the consistency you like.

Nutrition:

Calories: 115, Fat: 2 g, Carbs: 22 g, Protein: 4 g

4. Baby Kale Pineapple Smoothie

Preparation Time: **5 minutes**

Cooking Time: **5 minutes**

Servings: **2**

Ingredients:

- 1 cup almond milk

- 1/2 cup frozen pineapple

- 1 cup Kale

- 1 tablespoon hemp protein powder

Directions:

1. Place the almond milk, pineapple, and greens in the blender and blend until smooth.

2. Enjoy immediately.

Nutrition:

Calories: 185, Fat: 8 g, Carbs: 25 g, Protein: 8 g

5. Strawberry Coconut Smoothie

Preparation Time: **5 minutes**

Cooking Time: **5 minutes**

Servings: **2**

Ingredients:

- 1 cup coconut milk

- 1 frozen banana, sliced

- 2 cups frozen strawberries

- 1 teaspoon vanilla extract

- 1 tablespoon hemp protein powder

Directions:

1. Add all ingredients to the blender and blend until smooth.

2. Serve with ice.

Nutrition:

Calories: 165, Fat: 5 g, Carbs: 20 g, Protein: 11 g

6. Blueberry Bonanza Smoothies

Preparation Time: **5 minutes**

Cooking Time: **5 minutes**

Servings: **2**

Ingredients:

- 1/4 cup canned coconut or almond milk
- 1/2 cup water
- 1 medium banana, sliced
- 1 cup frozen blueberries
- 1 tablespoon raw almonds

Directions:

1. Add coconut milk, water, banana, blueberries and almonds to blender container.

2. Cover and blend until smooth. Pour into 2 glasses.

Nutrition:

Calories: 163, Fat: 1 g, Carbs: 30 g, Protein: 8 g

7. Peach Coconut Smoothie

Preparation Time: **5 minutes**

Cooking Time: **5 minutes**

Servings: **2**

Ingredients:

- 1 cup full fat coconut milk, chilled
- 1 cup ice
- 2 large fresh peaches, peeled and cut into chunks
- fresh lemon zest, to taste
- 1 tablespoon hemp protein powder

Directions:

1. Add coconut milk, ice and peaches blender. Using a zester, add a few gratings of fresh lemon zest.

2. Blend on high speed until smooth.

Nutrition:

Calories: 200, Fat: 5 g, Carbs: 35 g, Protein: 9 g

8. Key Lime Pie Smoothie

Preparation Time: **5 minutes**

Cooking Time: **5 minutes**

Servings: **2**

Ingredients:

- 1 cup coconut milk
- 1 cup ice
- 1/2 avocado
- zest and juice of 2 limes
- Pure liquid stevia to taste
- 1 tablespoon hemp protein powder

Directions:

1. Add all ingredients to the blender and blend until smooth.
2. Add ice and serve

Nutrition:

Calories: 200, Fat: 1 g, Carbs: 25 g, Protein: 20 g

9. High Protein and Nutritional Delish Smoothie

Preparation Time: **5 minutes**

Cooking Time: **5 minutes**

Servings: **2**

Ingredients:

- 1 cup almond milk
- 1/2 Avocado
- 4 Strawberries
- 1/2 Bananas (Very ripe)
- 1/2 cup Raw Kale or spinach
- 1/4 cup Carrot or 100 % Orange Juice
- 1 cup Coconut Yogurt or almond milk
- 1 tablespoon hemp protein powder

Directions:

1. Add ingredients to your blender and blend.
2. More water or ice can be added to help with your preferred texture/thickness.

Nutrition:

Calories: 250, Fat: 7 g, Carbs: 23 g, Protein: 25 g

10. Pineapple Protein Smoothie

Preparation Time: **5 minutes**

Cooking Time: **5 minutes**

Servings: **2**

Ingredients:

- 1 cup pineapple chunks
- 1 cup coconut milk (fresh or tinned)
- ½ med banana
- ¼ cup ice cubes
- ¼ tsp vanilla bean powder
- pinch low sodium salt
- 1 tablespoon hemp protein powder

Directions:

1. Peel pineapple and chop into small chunks.
2. Put everything into a high-speed blender and blend until smooth.

Nutrition:

Calories: 210, Fat: 2 g, Carbs: 25 g, Protein: 23 g

11. Raspberry Coconut Smoothie

Preparation Time: **5 minutes**

Cooking Time: **5 minutes**

Servings: **2**

Ingredients:

- ½ - 1 cup coconut milk (depending on how thick you like it)
- 1 medium banana, peeled sliced and frozen
- 2 teaspoons coconut extract (optional)
- 1 cup frozen raspberries
- 1 tablespoon hemp protein powder
- optional: shredded coconut flakes, and stevia to taste

Directions:

1. Add coconut milk, frozen banana slices and coconut extract to your blender.

2. Pulse 1-2 minutes until smooth.

3. Add frozen raspberries and continue to pulse until smooth.

4. Pour into your serving glass, top with a couple of raspberries and a little shredded coconut and enjoy!

Nutrition:

Calories: 160, Fat: 8 g, Carbs: 20 g, Protein: 2 g

12. Avocado Spinach Yogurt

Preparation Time: **5 minutes**

Cooking Time: **5 minutes**

Servings: **2**

Ingredients:

- 1 peeled and mashed ripe avocado
- 2 kiwis peeled and chopped
- 1 cup baby spinach, chopped
- 1 cup orange juice
- 1 cup vanilla Greek yogurt

Directions:

1. Mix all ingredients in blender and process till smooth.
2. Serve over crushed ice in tall glasses.
3. Makes 2 servings.

Nutrition:

Calories: 145, Fat: 1 g, Carbs: 13 g, Protein: 5 g

13. Cinnamon Banana and Broccoli

Preparation Time: **5 minutes**

Cooking Time: **5 minutes**

Servings: **2**

Ingredients:

- 2 teaspoons ground cinnamon
- 2 organic frozen bananas
- 3 cups almond milk
- 1/2 cup broccoli florets
- 2 tablespoons honey

Directions:

1. Prepare all ingredients in blender and mix until smooth.
2. Serve over crushed ice in tall glasses.
3. Makes 2 servings.

Nutrition:

Calories: 260, Fat: 1 g, Carbs: 58 g, Protein: 9 g

14. Coconut Grapes and Spinach

Preparation Time: **5 minutes**

Cooking Time: **5 minutes**

Servings: **2**

Ingredients:

- 1 cup seedless green grapes, frozen
- 2 cups spinach, chopped
- 2 frozen bananas
- 2 green apples peeled and sliced into small chunks
- 3 cups coconut water
- 2 teaspoons coconut oil
- 3 tablespoons honey
- 2 teaspoons ground flax seed

Directions:

1. Mix all ingredients into the blender.

2. Serve over crushed ice in tall glasses.

3. Makes 2 servings.

Nutrition:

Calories: 160, Fat: 0.4 g, Carbs: 38 g, Protein: 3 g

15. Lemon Blueberries and Spinach

Preparation Time: **5 minutes**

Cooking Time: **5 minutes**

Servings: **2**

Ingredients:

- 2 tablespoons lemon juice
- 1/2 cup blueberries fresh
- 1/2 cup strawberries fresh
- 1 banana peeled and sliced
- 1 1/2 cups baby spinach, chopped
- 1 tablespoon fresh mint
- Ice cubes

Directions:

1. Combine all ingredients except for ice cubes, and blend.
2. Add in ice cubes, and process till smooth.
3. Pour into tall glasses.
4. Makes 2 servings.

Nutrition:

Calories: 202, Fat: 1 g, Carbs: 47 g, Protein: 4 g

16. Lime Coconut with Spinach

Preparation Time: **5 minutes**

Cooking Time: **5 minutes**

Servings: **2**

Ingredients:

- 2 limes juiced
- 2 cups spinach, chopped
- 1 cup coconut milk
- 1 cup coconut water
- Ice cubes

Directions:

1. Mix all ingredients except for ice cubes and blend.

2. Add in ice cubes, and process till smooth.

3. Pour into tall glasses. Makes 2 servings.

Nutrition:

Calories: 185, Fat: 2 g, Carbs: 40 g, Protein: 8 g

17. Peach Kale Vanilla

Preparation Time: **5 minutes**

Cooking Time: **5 minutes**

Servings: **2**

Ingredients:

- 2 cups frozen peaches
- 3 cups kale chopped
- 2 scoops vanilla protein powder
- 2 cups unsweetened almond milk
- 1 cup frozen pineapple
- 1 banana peeled and sliced
- 2 tablespoons ground flax seed

Directions:

1. Combine all ingredients and blend till smooth.

2. Serve over crushed ice into tall glasses.

3. Makes 2 servings.

Nutrition:

Calories: 250, Fat: 5 g, Carbs: 39 g, Protein: 18 g

18. Pineapple Kale Banana

Preparation Time: **5 minutes**

Cooking Time: **5 minutes**

Servings: **2**

Ingredients:

- 1 3/4 cup chopped pineapple
- 2 1/4 cups chopped kale
- 3/4 cup coconut milk
- 1 1/2 bananas peeled and chopped
- Ice cubes

Directions:

1. Place all ingredients together except for ice cubes in the blender. Process till smooth.

2. Add ice cubes, and blend.

3. Pour into tall glasses. Makes 2 servings.

Nutrition:

Calories: 250, Fat: 4 g, Carbs: 50 g, Protein: 9 g

19. Raspberry Kale with Parsley

Preparation Time: **5 minutes**

Cooking Time: **5 minutes**

Servings: **2**

Ingredients:

- 1 1/4 cups organic frozen raspberries
- 1/2 cup chopped kale leaves
- 3/4 cup flat leaf parsley
- 1 1/2 bananas peeled and sliced
- 1 1/4 cup water
- 1 1/4 teaspoon ground flaxseed

Directions:

1. Mix all ingredients in blender, and process till smooth.
2. If the mixture is too thick, add additional water.
3. Serve over crushed ice in tall glasses.
4. Makes 2 servings.

Nutrition:

Calories: 150, Fat: 1 g, Carbs: 37 g, Protein: 3 g

CHAPTER 15

MAINS RECIPES

1. Pan-Fried Tilapia

Preparation Time: **10 minutes**

Cooking Time: **5-10 minutes**

Servings: **2**

Ingredients:

- ½ cup corn-starch or almond flour
- ½ teaspoon onion powder
- ½ teaspoon garlic powder
- ¼ teaspoon ground cumin
- ½ teaspoon chili powder
- 2 tilapia fillets (6 ounces each)
- Freshly ground pepper to taste
- Salt to taste
- 1 tablespoon fresh cilantro leaves, to garnish
- ½ tablespoon canola oil or vegetable oil

- Lime wedges to serve

1. Prepare all the dry ingredients into a bowl and stir.

2. Sprinkle salt and pepper over the fillets.

3. Put the fillets in the dry ingredients mixture. Shake to drop off extra mixture and place it on a plate.

4. Place a nonstick skillet over medium heat. Add oil. Add fillets and cook until the underside is golden brown.

5. Serve garnished with cilantro and with lime wedges.

Nutrition:

Calories: 210, Fat: 8 g, Carbs: 9 g, Protein: 22 g

2. Stir-Fried Pork with Ginger and Soy Sauce

Preparation Time: **15 minutes**

Cooking Time: **20 minutes**

Servings: **4**

Ingredients:

- 18 ounces pork tenderloin, trimmed of fat, chopped into bite size pieces
- 4 tablespoons dark soy sauce
- 11 ounces button mushrooms, sliced
- 5 ounces mange tout, trimmed
- 2 cloves garlic, peeled, thinly sliced
- Freshly ground pepper to taste
- 2 teaspoons corn-starch
- ¼ cup water
- 4 red bell peppers, deseeded, sliced
- 2 inches ginger, peeled, cut into thin matchsticks
- 8 spring onions, cut into 1-inch pieces

Directions:

1. Add some salt and pepper over pork and place it in the heated pan.
2. Cook until browned all over.
3. Add mushrooms and peppers and sauté for a couple of minutes.
4. Stir in mange tout and sauté for a minute.

5. Put in garlic, ginger and spring onions and cook until aromatic.

6. Add pork back into the pot.

7. Whisk together cornstarch, soy sauce and water in a bowl and pour into the wok.

8. Stir constantly until mixture thickens. Cook until the pork is cooked to the desired doneness.

9. Serve.

Nutrition:

Calories: 320, Fat: 29 g, Carbs: 2 g, Protein: 9 g

3. Harvest Chicken Casserole

Preparation Time: **15 minutes**

Cooking Time: **25 minutes**

Servings: **3**

Ingredients:

- 1 tablespoon extra-virgin olive oil + extra to grease
- Kosher salt to taste
- 1 small onion, chopped
- ½ pound Brussels sprouts, trimmed, quartered
- 1-pound skinless, boneless chicken breasts
- Freshly ground pepper to taste
- 1 medium sweet potato
- ½ teaspoon dried thyme
- 2 tablespoons chicken broth
- ¼ cup dried cranberries
- ½ teaspoon dried thyme
- 3 cups cooked wild rice
- ¼ cup sliced almonds

Directions:

1. Place a deep skillet over medium-high heat.
2. Add salt and pepper over the chicken and place it in the skillet.
3. Cook until golden.

4. Get with a slotted spoon and place it on your cutting board. Chop into bite size pieces.

5. Add sweet potato, onion and Brussels sprouts and stir.

6. Stir in thyme, salt, paprika and pepper and cook until soft.

7. Add in the broth and cover with a lid. Cook until sweet potato is soft.

8. Add rice, cranberries and chicken and mix well. Transfer into a greased baking dish. Sprinkle almonds on top.

9. Preheat oven at 325° F and bake for 20 minutes.

10. Let it cool for 5 minutes.

11. Serve.

Nutrition:

Calories: 1594, Fat: 21g, Carbs: 275g, Protein: 80g

4. Blackened Shrimp Bowls

Preparation Time: **10 minutes**

Cooking Time: **25 minutes**

Servings: **2**

Ingredients:

- ½ pound shrimp, discard tails, peeled, deveined
- ½ teaspoon paprika
- 1 teaspoon onion powder
- Freshly ground pepper to taste
- ½ cup fire roasted corn
- 1 tablespoon chopped cilantro + extra to garnish
- 1 small avocado, peeled, pitted, sliced
- 1 cup cooked brown rice
- 1 teaspoon ground cumin
- ½ teaspoon garlic powder
- Kosher salt to taste
- 1 tablespoon olive oil, divided
- ½ red pepper, diced
- Juice of ½ lime, divided

Directions:

For shrimp:

1. Add shrimp into a bowl. Sprinkle all the spices and salt over it. Toss well.

2. Place a skillet over medium-high heat. Add half the oil.

3. Add shrimp and cook until it turns translucent.

For salad:

4. Add corn, red pepper and cilantro into a bowl and toss.

5. Drizzle remaining oil, lime juice, salt and pepper over it and toss well.

6. Add ½ cup rice into each bowl. Layer with shrimp followed by corn salad and finally avocado slices.

7. Sprinkle cilantro on top and drizzle lime juice and serve.

Nutrition:

Calories: 380, Fat: 8 g, Carbs: 39 g, Protein: 40 g

5. No-Chop Skillet Chili

Preparation Time: **15 minutes**

Cooking Time: **45 minutes**

Servings: **4**

Ingredients:

- 2 teaspoons canola oil
- 2 cans unsalted red kidney beans, rinsed, drained
- 2 packages frozen sweet pepper and onion stir-fry vegetables
- 4-6 teaspoons chili powder
- 24 ounces lean ground beef
- 2 cans unsalted diced tomatoes, with its liquid
- 2 packages low sodium taco seasoning or chili seasoning
- 4 tablespoons ketchup
- To serve: Use any one or more
- Low fat shredded Cheddar cheese
- Black olives, sliced
- Plain fat free Greek yogurt
- Green onions, sliced
- Chopped cilantro

Directions:

1. Prepare a cast iron skillet over high heat. Add beef and sauté until brown.

2. Add rest of the ingredients except ketchup then stir.

3. Lower the heat and cover with a lid. Simmer until the vegetables are cooked.

4. Turn off the heat. Add ketchup and stir.

5. Let it rest for a while with cover.

6. Ladle into bowls. Top with the suggested toppings and serve.

Nutrition:

Calories: 290, Fat: 6 g, Carbs: 32 g, Protein: 25 g

6. Turmeric Chicken Stew

Preparation Time: **15 minutes**

Cooking Time: **30 minutes**

Servings: **3**

Ingredients:

- 1 tablespoon olive oil
- 1 sweet potato, cubed
- 1 medium eggplant, cubed
- ½ tablespoon minced fresh ginger
- ¼ cup low sodium chicken broth
- 1 chicken breast, skinless, boneless, cubed
- 1 small red onion, chopped
- 1 clove garlic, minced
- 1 teaspoon turmeric powder

Directions:

1. Place a skillet over medium-high heat. Add oil.

2. Put chicken and sear until browned.

3. Stir in the onion and sweet potato and cook until onion turns pink.

4. Stir in garlic, eggplant, ginger and turmeric and sauté for a few seconds until aromatic.

5. Add broth and simmer until the desired thickness is achieved. Stir occasionally.

6. Ladle into bowls and serve.

Calories: 185, Fat: 5 g, Carbs: 24 g, Protein: 10 g

7. Warm Chicken Salad

Preparation Time: **10 minutes**

Cooking Time: **15 minutes**

Servings: **4**

Ingredients:

- 4 small chicken breasts, skinless, boneless, halved
- 2 large orange or red bell pepper, deseeded, cut into 1-inch squares
- 3 1/2 ounces watercress, discard hard stalks
- 1 medium cucumber, sliced
- 2 little gem lettuce, leaves separated
- 4 medium tomatoes, chopped
- 2 tsp. thick balsamic vinegar
- Sea salt to taste
- Freshly ground pepper to taste

Directions:

1. Sprinkle salt and pepper over the chicken.

2. Prepare a large nonstick pan over high heat. Spray with cooking spray.

3. Add chicken and cook until light brown all over. Remove onto your chopping board. Cook in batches if required. Spray the pan in each batch.

4. Let it cool and cut into slices.

5. Spray some oil in the pan. Add bell pepper and cook until slightly

charred. Turn off the heat.

6. Place watercress, tomatoes and cucumber over the lettuce.

7. Scatter the cooked bell pepper. Place chicken slices all over.

8. Put balsamic vinegar and lemon juice on top. Sprinkle pepper on top and serve.

Nutrition:

Calories: 260, Fat: 10 g, Carbs: 18 g, Protein: 18 g

8. White Bean Wrap

Preparation Time: **15 minutes**

Cooking Time: **15 minutes**

Servings: **2**

Ingredients:

- 1 tablespoon apple cider vinegar
- 1 teaspoon finely chopped canned chipotle chili in adobo sauce
- 1 cup shredded red cabbage
- 2 tablespoons chopped fresh cilantro
- 1 small ripe avocado, peeled, pitted, chopped
- 1 tablespoon minced red onion
- ½ tablespoon canola oil
- Salt to taste
- 1 small carrot, shredded
- ½ can white beans, rinsed
- ¼ cup shredded Sharp Cheddar cheese
- 2 whole wheat wraps or tortillas (8-10 inches each)

Directions:

1. Add vinegar, chipotle chili, oil and salt into a bowl and whisk well.

2. Add the vegetables and toss well.

3. Add beans and avocado into another bowl and mash until desired consistency.

4. Put cheese and onion and mix well.

5. Spread about ½ cup of the bean mixture on the wraps. Scatter cabbage mixture.

6. Wrap in foil if desired and serve.

Nutrition:

Calories: 340, Fat: 15 g, Carbs: 44 g, Protein: 12 g

9. Broccoli, Beef & Potato Hot Dish w

Preparation Time: **20 minutes**

Cooking Time: **1 hour**

Servings: **4**

Ingredients:

- 3/4-pound broccoli, cut into 1-inch florets
- 3/4-pound lean ground beef
- Salt to taste
- Worcestershire sauce
- 3 tablespoons corn-starch
- 1/8 teaspoon turmeric powder
- 1 small egg, lightly beaten
- 1/8 teaspoon paprika
- 1 tablespoon canola oil
- 1 medium onion, chopped
- ½ tsp. garlic powder
- 2 cups low-fat milk
- Freshly ground pepper to taste
- 1 cup shredded Sharp Cheddar cheese
- 2 cups frozen hash-brown or precooked shredded potatoes

Directions:

1. Place broccoli in a bowl. Drizzle ½ tablespoon oil over it.

2. Toss well and transfer onto a baking sheet. Spread it in a single layer.

3. Preheated oven at 450° F for about 15-20 minutes or brown at a few places.

4. Add remaining oil into the skillet.

5. Put beef and onion then cook until brown.

6. Add Worcestershire sauce, salt and garlic powder and mix well. Turn off the heat and transfer into a baking dish.

7. Add milk and cornstarch into a saucepan and whisk well. Place saucepan over medium-high heat.

8. Stir constantly until thick. Add Cheddar cheese, turmeric and salt and mix well. Stir constantly until cheese melts.

9. Pour cheese sauce over the beef mixture. Scatter broccoli on top.

10. Add egg, hash-browns, salt and pepper into a bowl and mix well. Spread it over the broccoli. Spray with cooking spray.

11. Preheat oven at 400° F and bake for 20-30 minutes or brown at a few places.

12. Take from the oven and garnish with paprika.

13. Cool for 10 minutes and serve.

Nutrition:

Calories: 410, Fat: 19 g, Carbs: 25 g, Protein: 30 g

10. Cheddar-Stuffed Mini Meatloaves with Chipotle Glaze

Preparation Time: **15 minutes**

Cooking Time: **40 minutes**

Servings: **2**

Ingredients:

- ½ pound lean ground beef
- 3 tablespoons fine, dry whole-wheat breadcrumbs
- 3 tablespoons ketchup
- ½ teaspoon ground cumin
- Freshly ground pepper to taste
- 1/8 teaspoon ground chipotle pepper
- 1 small onion, finely chopped
- 1 small egg
- 1 teaspoon chili powder
- Salt to taste
- ¼ cup shredded extra-sharp Cheddar cheese

Directions:

1. Grease 2 small baking dishes or mini loaf pans with cooking spray. Place them on a baking sheet.

2. Set aside cheese, chipotle chili and 2 tablespoons of ketchup and add rest of the ingredients into a bowl. Mix well.

3. Divide equally and place in the prepared pans. Using your finger, make a deep cut of about 1-½ inches along the central line on top of the meatloaves.

4. Sprinkle cheese a tablespoon of cheese in this indentation in each of the meatloaves. Press the edges of the cuts together so that the cheese remains stuffed in the meatloaves.

5. Add chipotle chili and 2 tablespoons ketchup into a bowl and stir. Brush this mixture on top of the meatloaves.

6. Place the meatloaves along with the baking sheet in a preheated oven.

7. Bake at 450° F for 20-30 minutes or until a meat thermometer when inserted in the center of the meatloaves shows 165° F.

8. Serve warm.

Nutrition:

Calories: 380, Fat: 7 g, Carbs: 18 g, Protein: 37 g

CHAPTER 16

OTHER TYPES OF INTERMITTENT FASTING

Choosing the right diet for you will depend on a few things. You need to consider what you are trying to gain from Intermittent Fasting. So, you want to see which of these adaptations is optimal for achieving those particular goals. Pay attention to any considerations you might have.

If you decide that the one you have chosen does not suit your needs or you feel too demanding to maintain after some trial or error, consider trying a different adaptation. However, be sure to give everyone an effort of at least a few weeks to ensure that the challenges are not simply getting used to your new diet.

12 Hours of Fasting

The average person fasts for about eight hours each night. So, the 12-hour fast is not very far from what you probably already do naturally in your daily life. When you follow the 12-hour fasting diet, you want to maintain the same fasting duration and eat windows every day.

Completing the 12-hour fast diet should not require too much adaptation to your regular food routine. Chances are you've already eaten close enough to this type of program in your daily life, however. The biggest adjustment to this type of fasting is that you have to eliminate late-night snacks. Late-night snacking tends to be the primary way people consume food between 19:00 and 7:00, however. Letting go of this habit can help you deal with Intermittent Fasting cycles and get many benefits without drastic changes.

Another reason why this diet may be easier for beginners is that you still have much time to eat the same number of calories per day than you are used to. Other diets with shorter dietary windows generally don't allow you enough time to eat as many calories in your day, leading to a transition phase as you get used to your new food cycles.

12-hour fasting is an excellent practice for those who have just started with Intermittent Fasting. Alternatively, it may be a better consideration for those who cannot engage in a more intense diet variation for health reasons. It is easy to adapt and can support you in maintaining any other dietary needs that you may have to consider since it does not require any substantial changes to your current eating habits.

Skipping Meals

Skipping meals is an extremely flexible form of Intermittent Fasting, which can provide all the benefits of Intermittent Fasting but with less rigid planning. If you are not someone who has a typical schedule or feels like a more rigorous variation of the Intermittent Fasting diet will serve you, skipping meals is viable.

Many people who choose to use skipped meals find that it is a great way to listen to their bodies and follow their basic instincts. If they are not hungry, they don't eat that meal. Instead, they wait for others. Skipping meals can also help people who have time constraints and may not always be able to eat a specific meal.

The best way to successfully skip meals is to learn to stay in tune with your body and focus on what you need. Often, people find that they aren't hungry 3+ times a day. So instead of eating several meals, they only eat when they are hungry.

It is essential to realize that skipping meals may not always be possible to maintain a 10-16 hour fasting window. You may not get all the benefits of other fasting diets. However, this could be an excellent solution for an Intermittent Fasting diet that feels more natural. It could also be a great idea for those looking to start listening to their bodies more so that they can adapt to more intense diet variation more easily. It can be an excellent transition diet for you if you are not ready to jump into one of the other fasting diets.

Warrior Diet Fasting

The most extreme form of Intermittent Fasting is known as the warrior diet. This Intermittent Fasting cycle follows a 20-hour fasting window with a short 4-hour consumption window. During that eating window, individuals should consume only raw fruits and vegetables. They can also eat a big meal. Typically, the window for eating occurs at night, so people can snack during the evening, eat a big meal, and then resume fasting.

Due to the length of the fast that takes place during the warrior's diet, people should also consume a relatively abundant level of healthy fats. In this way, you will give the body something to consume during the fast with which to produce energy. A small number of carbohydrates can also be incorporated to support energy levels.

People who eat the warrior diet tend to believe that humans are natural night eaters and that we are not meant to eat during the day. The belief is that eating in this way follows our natural circadian rhythms, allowing our body to work optimally.

The only people who should consider following the warrior's diet have already had success with other forms of Intermittent Fasting and are used to it. Attempting to jump directly into the warrior's diet can have severe repercussions for anyone unaccustomed to Intermittent Fasting. Even still, those used to it may find this particular style too extreme to be maintained.

It is essential that if you follow the warrior's diet, be very careful about your health. You may find that you are malnourished or struggle with other health problems if you are not careful. These health problems are counterintuitive and increase the risk of contracting diseases like cancer rather than decreasing it.

Those who have learned to eat according to the ways of the Warrior Diet become accustomed to claiming to be in excellent health. They tend to have excellent energy levels, minimal fat deposits, and healthier systems in general. That is if they are keeping their nourishment within that 4-hour food window—those who have not experienced great success with this diet and often find it challenging to maintain it.

Alternate Days

Alternating the day on which you fast are a common variation of the Intermittent Fasting diet. It also happens to have many of its unique adaptations. Typically, what you choose is based on what makes you feel better and helps you get the best results.

Some people choose to completely avoid solid foods on their fasting days, while others will eat up to 500 calories. On days when the individual usually eats, they can eat as much as they want. This is an extreme version of the Intermittent Fasting diet, and more work may be needed to acclimate your body to this dietary habit so you can properly maintain it. You could also start eating up to 500 calories and then reduce to not having solids on fasting days, or you could stay with 500 calories days.

Studies have shown that alternating fasting days is effective in supporting people with their heart health. It is also an incredible variation for people who want to lose weight. A study conducted found that the average person lost around 11 pounds over 12 weeks using this diet.

Due to how extreme this fasting diet can be, it is not ideal for anyone who has never fasted before. Even if you have fasted naturally for quite long periods, you should first work to intentionally support a more relaxed variation of the Intermittent Fasting diet before moving on to alternate days. You should also avoid this fasting style if you are dealing with certain medical conditions as it can harm you. If you consider the diet on alternate days for Intermittent Fasting, be sure to let your doctor know about your specific plans. This can help them determine what the right decision would be to avoid negative health impacts.

CHAPTER 17

WHAT TO EAT WHILE INTERMITTENT FASTING

There are some of the foods that you simply must include in your diet while you take up the fast.

Water

This is the essential element to consume when you take up the intermittent fast. Water can act as an elixir when it comes to losing weight. You must keep your body hydrated and ensure that all the toxins are dissolved and eliminated. All your organs need water to remain fresh and healthy; right from your liver to gut, to digestive tracts, water helps keep these organs working smoothly.

Drink at least 8 - 10 glasses of water a day and focus more on the fasting period. You can consume water with fruit. This refers to water that has fruit and herbs infused into it. Fill up a jar with water and toss in fruit and herbs such as oranges, lemons, mint leaves, and a cinnamon dash. Consume this every few hours. Remember that the intermittent fast can be quite taxing and lead to side effects such as headaches and nausea. In such a case, only water can help you out and put an end to these.

Fish

Fish can be considered as a miracle food as it can significantly help with weight loss. According to dietary guidelines, people need to consume at least 6 to 8 ounces of fish every week. Fish contains a lot of nutrients. It is rich in fats, proteins and Vitamin D. This means you do not have to worry about denying your body these nutrients by taking on the fast. You do not have to reach for supplements if you can consume fish regularly. Fish is also rich in DHA, which helps in brain development. You will see that your mind is fresher, and you can think well. Your productivity will increase, and stress will be curbed.

Avocado

You might wonder why avocado is on this list, considering it is one of the fattiest foods. However, you must understand that the fasting phase can take a toll on your body and consume foods that keep you going. It is rich in monounsaturated fat, which is great for those who tend to get hungry quite fast. It keeps you feeling full for longer. You will not find yourself reaching out to eat a snack. Avocado is quite versatile and can be added to your breakfast or lunch menu. Those who tend to include it in their breakfast menu can generally go without food for longer periods without complaining about hunger.

Leafy Greens

Leafy green vegetables are loaded with multiple nutrients that are great for your body. These include the likes of kale, broccoli, lettuce, etc. These are loaded with fiber. Fiber keeps your body going when you suffer from digestive issues such as constipation. You are sure to go through it when you adopt the intermittent fast. In such a case, it becomes that much more important to consume these vegetables to keep your stomach in good shape. Fiber also makes you feel fuller and not feel too hungry between meals.

Potatoes

Potatoes are rich in carbs that can keep you sated for hours. Make sure you either steam and mash them or roast them without any oil or fat. Deep frying them is never an option. You can consume them with their skin on as it contains a lot of nutrition.

Probiotics

When it comes to digestion, both your liver and gut play a vital role. Both of them need a healthy dose of probiotics to function optimally. If you have an unhealthy gut, you might suffer from side effects such as constipation and even leaky gut syndrome. To combat these is by consuming as many probiotics as possible. Some natural foods rich in probiotics include kombucha and kefir. Add these to your meals, and you are sure to experience positive benefits. An alternative is to go for probiotic supplements. Make sure you know which ones to go for. You can consult a physician first.

Assorted Berries

There is nothing better than consuming fresh berries in the mornings. They are loaded with antioxidants and vital nutrients required to keep your body healthy. Strawberries, raspberries, blueberries, and gooseberries are all great for you. Place them into the blender with some milk or yogurt to make a smoothie. According to studies, those who consumed berries regularly stayed within their ideal body weight and did not gain too much weight over longer periods.

Eggs

An essential aspect of losing weight is building lean muscles. Lean muscles replace regular ones and prevent fat from getting stored. You can build lean muscle by consuming foods rich in proteins. One important source of protein is eggs. Those who consume eggs for breakfast are better positioned to develop lean muscles and not go hungry before the next meal. Eggs can be quite versatile and cooked in any way you like. Hard-boil them the previous day so that you have a ready meal the following day. Simply toss them in a pan to scramble them. It only takes a few minutes to cook them.

Whole Grains

One aspect of maintaining a clean and healthy diet is going for whole grains. The intermittent fast promotes consumption of these, as they are easier for the body to digest and keep the system clean. They are also loaded with proteins and fiber. Do not limit yourself to the usual such as wheat and oats and go for something different such as Bulgar, amaranth, and flax.

Nuts

Nuts are fatty, but they contain good fat. Not all fat is bad fat as there can be some good fat as well. Polyunsaturated fats are said to be good for the body and can keep you feeling full for longer. You will not feel hungry if you munch on some walnuts or almonds. But make sure you make them a part of your meal and do not snack on them. Snacking on them can leave you feeling full and disrupt your meal plan. Do not worry about the calorie aspect. Nuts are not as calorific as you may have thought. They contain far fewer calories than some of the other fatty foods that people tend to snack on.

These happen to be superfoods that you must include in your diet while you take up Intermittent Fasting.

Foods to Avoid While Intermittent Fasting

Processed foods

Processed foods include biscuits, wafers, chips, cakes, and sugary drinks such as cola. These will only add to your distresses and counteract your weight loss goals. Try to avoid these at all costs.

Junk foods

Make it a point to avoid all junk food from your diet. There should be no room for burgers, pizzas, and pasta that contain a lot of fat.

Although wine is said to be quite healthy, it would be best to limit it to just 1 serving per week. Try your best to avoid consuming hard liquor.

With Intermittent Fasting, many people tend to follow their usual eating habits in terms of the specific foods that they put on their plate during each meal. They expect that they will lose weight just because they have fasted during the morning, night, and afternoon.

Just as there are many foods that you can surely include in your diet to help you lose that extra weight that is causing you concern, there are also some foods that you should always try to avoid if your goal is to lose weight.

CHAPTER 18

INTERMITTENT FASTING AND WEIGHT LOSS

Weight loss benefits can be derived from Intermittent Fasting. We have established how any Intermittent Fasting methods can lead you to lose weight and keep it off. The primary reason why most people engage in Intermittent Fasting is to lose weight and feel better about themselves. You can expand your weight loss potential by following some simple but effective guidelines.

Cause of Weight Gain and Obesity

Your regular diet plays a critical role in holding you back in your weight loss endeavors. A high-fat, high sugar diet will only lead you to gain weight and increase difficulty in shedding those extra pounds. Also, you might even be experiencing some health issues, as well.

The main reason you are packing on the pounds is not so much in the number of calories you are consuming as derived from sugar, fats, and carbs, but it is the fact that your body becomes overloaded with them. This overload causes your body to fall behind and become unable to process all of these substances.

After a certain period, they become toxic in your body and may cause you to become intoxicated. This intoxication can become manifest in any number of ways and can cause any number of results.

For instance, you might become intoxicated with high levels of sugar in your system. In addition to having high blood sugar, which is a precursor to diabetes, you might have trouble sleeping, getting skin rashes, and even having blurry vision. These are some of the symptoms of high levels of blood sugar.

But what having such high levels of blood sugar does to your body is cause you to become intoxicated to a point where both your digestive system and your metabolism cannot work fast to keep up with the rush calories. This is especially true if you are eating all day long or if you binge. Since your body is unable to keep up, your digestive system will find the best way to cope. In that sense, your digestive system may begin to stop breaking down foods into nutrients and send them straight to the liver.

When this happens, you begin to develop a condition known as "fatty liver." When you eventually have a fatty liver, your digestive system is essentially unable to process any foods. So, what the body does is send them straight to the fat stores.

Most people don't realize that you could be consuming even more calories from drinks than you could be from food. Drinks such as sugary sodas and fruit drinks will wreak havoc on your metabolism. Also, energy and sports drinks will do a number on your body as well. These are generally high in various types of chemicals or may contain artificial sweeteners, some of which have been deemed unsafe for human consumption.

These sports and energy drinks may give you temporary boosts in energy and concentration but only serve to intoxicate your body. A good sign of this intoxication is when you need to consume an ever-increasing amount of these drinks to achieve the same results.

We have indicated that the Intermittent Fasting approach does not call for the restriction of any foods in any way. It does call for the moderation of food portions and the implementation of a balanced diet.

An increased amount of fruits, vegetables, lean proteins, whole grains, fiber, and healthy fats are essential building blocks of a healthy lifestyle. It is recommended that you begin to look at how you can begin to shift eating habits on regular days so that you leave out much of the processed stuff and consume more fresh, wholesome stuff. This requires a pattern shift in your mindset about the foods you eat and their portions.

If you limit the size of the portions and the number of times you eat certain foods, you are already on your way to losing weight and keeping it off.

When you start by setting yourself up with a balanced diet during your regular days, your fasting days will be turbocharged. You will kick your weight loss habits into overdrive, and the weight will begin to come off.

Best of all, if you combine a solid diet with regular exercise, you will be well on your way to creating an incredibly fit and healthy version. This will enable you to process foods better, reverse some of the adverse conditions in your body, and help you regain confidence about the way you look and feel. These are just some of how you can benefit from losing weight through Intermittent Fasting.

The body can adapt to changes in caloric intake in such a way that the body will find the best ways to continue hoarding calories as per its hardwiring.

This is where Intermittent Fasting provides the opportunity to force the body to stay on its toes.

As we get older, more sedentary, and certainly overloading food consumption, the body packs on more and more calories. So, when you try to cut back on your consumption by reducing portions or just skipping meals, your body will quickly adapt to that and revert to its calorie-hoarding ways.

That is why Intermittent Fasting provides you with the opportunity to lose weight by mixing up your metabolism. The body continues consuming calories to keep the body humming along on all cylinders. As long as you don't starve yourself and trigger starvation mode, the body will begin to draw its reserves to the body strong.

When you fast, the body will consume whatever it has in the bloodstream, that is, the last intake of food you had before beginning your fasting period. When that happens, that intake eventually runs out, and the body needs to draw energy from somewhere. It will dip into its fat stores and convert body fat into glucose so it can be utilized as energy. You are beginning to use up body fat and make the most of your fasting period.

Things get dicey when you fast for too long and trigger starvation mode. When this happens, your body will begin to burn muscle rather than fat and cause you to lose weight.

When your metabolism gets faster, what you are doing makes your body process food faster and convert nutrients into energy before it is stored as fat in the body. If you fall into a routine, your body will adjust, and you will plateau. When you see that you are beginning to plateau, it's time to mix things up again. All you have to do is a plan for changes as you go along.

For example, you decide that your fasting days will be Monday and Thursday. After some time, this may become predictable for the body. So, you can plan to mix things up after two months and fast on Tuesdays and Saturdays.

The reason for a change is that you are switching up days and the time between those days. After the next two months, you can choose to fast on different days or go back to the last arrangement. In any case, you are proactively giving your body the runaround.

By mixing things up continuously, you will be ensuring that your body won't get the chance to adjust. You will become accustomed to your new eating plan. This will help you achieve your weight loss plans and help you keep the weight off.

Intermittent Fasting is an important way to improve your overall health, drop weight, and create a lifelong plan that will help you stay in shape and keep the pounds off. This new lifestyle begins with you having a shift in your mindset. Ensure to have a balanced diet as you possibly can.

You can devise your Intermittent Fasting plans by choosing any one of the methods we have described herein. Perhaps you are fond of transitioning from the 5:2 to the 16/8 to the Eat-stop-eat methods. Whichever way you choose to approach your Intermittent Fasting plans, you will begin to see the results in reducing your body fat, weight loss, and overall health improvement.

CHAPTER 19

INTERMITTENT FASTING TIPS FOR SUCCESS

While Intermittent Fasting is beneficial, it can be challenging to get started to the point where your body adjusts to a new schedule. There are some tips that can help set you on the path to success.

Have a Conversation With Yourself

Intermittent Fasting has a wide variety of proven benefits, but that does not mean it is for everyone. Before you attempt a fast, it is essential to have a real dialogue with yourself and consider your self-discipline, current attachment to food, and any regular activities that would make fasting difficult, your general lifestyle, and your level of exercise. Deciding to try a different fitness regime is a lot easier on day one than after struggling through a week or more of fasting.

Watch Your Response

While it is essential to keep tabs on how your body responds to Intermittent Fasting, it is doubly important to monitor your vitals during the initial phase when your body is adjusting to the new feeding times. Some discomfort is expected for the first three to four weeks. Anything longer or more should be discussed with a doctor as soon as possible.

The Early Days Will Have Ups and Downs

While your body adjusts to Intermittent Fasting, there will be times when you lose weight, and your body is trying to keep on to every calorie it has. This is natural and to be expected as your body realigns its hormone levels.

Drink Lots of Water

This doesn't mean stay hydrated, which is good advice regardless, it means to drink at minimum a gallon of water each day. It will help you feel full and ensure your body continues processing toxins normally, even if it is holding onto all of its fat due to the transition. This is a good exercise for most people anyway, as roughly 40 percent of adults are walking around right now in a mild state of dehydration. If thirst remains untreated for long enough, it starts manifesting itself as hunger, so staying hydrated will keep you feeling fuller longer in two ways.

Use Caffeine as a Tool

When you first begin training your body to expect food less often. Drinking black coffee or a zero-calorie soda every 3 or 4 hours can make it easier to get through the early fasts as caffeine is known to suppress the appetite actively. It is essential not to go overboard, as many artificial sweeteners have been known to cause health problems when consumed in large amounts. Also, it is important not to begin to rely on caffeine to the point that your body doesn't adapt to the fasting schedule. Feel free to use as much caffeine as you need to get through the first few days of fasting but keep your intake under control from there as you want your body to be building new habits, not simply have its appetite stunted by caffeine.

Don't Expect Constant Weight Loss

While you will likely see weight loss first as your body adapts to fewer calories in its system on average, this will probably start and stop throughout your time fasting. Especially after the first few weeks of the transition as your body tries to hold on to everything it has until it can figure out what is going on. Once it gets with the program, however, things should proceed as expected.

Every diet will have periods of weight loss plateau, which is simply a part of weight loss that cannot be mitigated. As long as you stay, consistent weight loss will eventually resume. The worst thing you can do is try and change things up to get weight loss back on track, as that will only make it more difficult for your body to start shedding weight once more.

Find Things to Do

When they begin fasting, the first instinct that many people have is to refrain from doing anything that isn't essential to prevent the loss of every possible calorie. Unfortunately, this is a terrible plan to put into action as the net benefit is negligible, and the mental anguish you put yourself through will far outweigh it anyway. This is because time spent doing nothing is time that, in practice, is going to be spent watching every second that ticks by in hopes of forcing the hour you can break your fast to appear.

As such, the trick to make the final few hours of any fast go by as quickly as possible is to find an activity that is not difficult but does require a reasonable amount of concentration. Doing so will help to ensure that you can eat again before you know it. It is also important to ensure that the task you choose is not too difficult, as your mind is likely not at its best at this point, but that it takes up enough of your attention that you stop paying attention to the hands of the clock.

Stick with low-intensity exercises: If you plan on exercising while fasting, you must limit your cardio to only low-intensity variety. This equates to a light jog or 10 minutes, as long as you aren't pushing yourself past your limits.

It is important to take the time to listen to the signals your body is giving and take a break if you feel immediately. If you ignore what your body is trying to tell you and attempt to power through, it will only make the rest of your workout seem unmanageable.

Up Your Protein Intake

Standard is that you want to take between 20 and 30 grams of protein every four hours while awake. While Intermittent Fasting makes this unattainable, you're still going to want to take between 80 and 120 grams of protein per day. If you plan a serious strength workout, you will want to do so between two snacks, if not two full meals.

Keep in mind that snacks are going to be your friend, as long as your Intermittent Fasting plan supports them. A snack or a meal consumed between 3 and 4 hours before a workout should be enough to keep your blood sugar up through a standard exercise, or between 1 and 2 hours if you are vulnerable to low blood sugar. These meals should include blood-sugar stabilizing protein and fast-acting carbs, such as two pieces of toast with banana slices and peanut butter. Sometime in the two hours after your workout, you will want to try and consume approximately 20 grams of protein and 20 grams of carbs to ensure maximum muscle growth and get your glycogen stores high enough to maintain energy until it is time to eat again.

Intermittent Fasting is a new phenomenon in the diet which is here to last. It has plenty of health benefits for your health and also for your mind every day. One of the reasons Intermittent Fasting is so successful is that there is less time to eat during the day. You eat just 6-8 hours with Intermittent Fasting, while most people do the reverse by eating 16-18 hours a day. Fasting is among the most ancient healing practices in human history observed by nearly every religion and culture on earth. Consumers all over the world realize that Intermittent Fasting will accelerate weight loss in ways that can't achieve calorie restriction on itself.

There is plenty of information to support the effects of Intermittent Fasting, but consumers are often suspicious regarding their health and are justifiably worried. But is it safe with Intermittent Fasting? The quick reply is yes. Intermittent Fasting is healthy unless you eat the right foods for your wellness and fitness objectives. Below, we break down the truth about how Intermittent Fasting may be used to support your health.

Most people adopt an Intermittent Fasting diet, and it's not an uncommon bio-hack. The primary reason people pursue Intermittent Fasting is weight loss. Yet Intermittent Fasting offers other benefits for the body. Fasting is moreover a daily part of cultural and religious practices. Intermittent Fasting is not about cutting off food entirely, missing meals or not eating for a risky amount of days in the end; it is about eating at certain times and not eating at other times, or eating in "cycles," as is often known. You're restricting calories with Intermittent Fasting where you eat different times of the day or on certain days. In a fasted cycle, you compensate for the lack of nutrients by improving your nutrients with other meals and potentially supplements over a period where you eat.

Intermittent Fasting isn't a diet based on calories, either. Low-calorie diets at first have a reputation for success, and then fail as the person begins to develop cravings. It isn't just about not eating either. It's more of an eating disorder and eating disorders of anorexia are a more severe problem – simply minimizing the food you consume may not make you healthier. As long as you eat the right foods for your health and fitness objectives by food or drink, Intermittent Fasting is perfectly healthy.

Although Intermittent Fasting is healthy, it is not a form of diet that we can all use. First and foremost, please speak to an advisor regarding Intermittent Fasting, particularly if you have identified medical problems before beginning your routine. If you're unclear whether Intermittent Fasting is appropriate for you, this list might point out explanations for maybe not doing it. If you have an eating disorder or previously had an eating disorder, it could be safer to stop Intermittent Fasting.

While Intermittent Fasting decreases insulin and can help avoid diabetes, it may not be a successful approach in certain situations. If you do have diabetes, it's better to speak to the doctor because the variations in type 1 and type 2 in your particular case may mean that you don't have the correct Intermittent Fasting.

Sometimes after you have met your goal for weight loss, it can be challenging to manage Intermittent Fasting. It doesn't have to be difficult to stick to your fasting-focused lifestyle, though. You have to have the right attitude and the proper routines in place, so you never give up, and you never undermine the results that you have achieved.